Infants and children

An introduction to emotional development

by

Mirabelle Maslin

Augur Press

INFANTS AND CHILDREN:
AN INTRODUCTION TO EMOTIONAL DEVELOPMENT
Copyright © Mirabelle Maslin 2013
The moral right of the author has been asserted

Author of: Beyond the Veil
Tracy
Carl and other writings
Fay
On a Dog Lead
Emily
The Fifth Key
The Candle Flame
The Supply Teacher's Surprise
Miranda
Lynne
Field Fare
Lentigo Maligna Melanoma

British Library Cataloguing in Publication Data.
A catalogue record for this book is available from
the British Library.

ISBN 978-0-9571380-2-5
First published 2013 by
Augur Press
Delf House
52 Penicuik Road
Roslin
Midlothian EH25 9LH
United Kingdom

Printed by Lightning Source

Infants and children

An introduction to emotional development

Dedication

To all children, born, and as yet unborn, and the child within each adult person in every race and creed.

To my daughter-in-law, Vanessa, who generously and lovingly does everything she can to foster secure emotional development in those children who come into her care. Without her, this book would not have been written. Her relentless and forceful but appropriate insistence about the crucial importance of this task has led to its timely completion.

To Dr Norman Taylor, psychiatrist, who has helped countless people during his working life, and beyond. His interest and encouragement during the writing of this book have been invaluable.

"All that people seem to want to know is whether my baby will be a girl or a boy. When it is born, no doubt they will remark upon who my baby reminds them of – mother, father, uncle, aunt…

"It seems that no one refers to the most important thing of all – the crucial task of discovering who this person truly is."

My daughter, at 30 weeks of pregnancy with her first baby.

Author's note:
I feel that the English language does not yet have adequate
vocabulary that embodies both male and female. Our society is
alert to the limitations of using only the male forms, but I ask
the reader to bear with me in the preponderance of 'he, him,
his, himself' versions when I refer to a child. Much of the
reason for this is the potentially cumbersome nature, and
possible confusion, inherent in referring to both Mother and
child using 'she/her/hers/herself'.

Introduction

Although the content of this book is primarily for parents and others who have responsibility for the care of children, it is of relevance to anyone. Every one of us was once a child, and every one of us had to undergo a process of development that was supervised by people of adult years.

When we struggle in our adult lives it is not uncommon to find that there is a resonance between current problems and difficulties that we encountered in early life. Understanding such links can aid us in the task of improving the outcome of present-day situations where difficult emotions are interfering with our capacity to deal with the matter in hand.

It is my hope that the material I have included in this book will help readers to expand their thinking. Any consequent evolution of their humanity will be of great benefit to the next generation.

This book is for 'grown-ups' to read about the care of children, but how might a child react to discovering that there was nothing in it *for him*? I have therefore included in the appendix a short story – *A Story of Tim* – that I wrote specifically for small children.

Contents

Preface

This book is not intended to be a comprehensive reference book for all eventualities, emotional or physical. No book could ever achieve such a goal, as human experience is so diverse and multifaceted that no one can work out an ideal formula for the dilemmas of each parent in relation to each child at any particular point in time.

One can predict with a certain amount of accuracy what the outcome of some situations may well be, but one can never be sure, as the development of the final result can be affected by factors of which we might at the time know nothing.

When Sleeping Beauty pricked her finger on a spindle, she would have died of the wound had not the twelfth fairy given the possibility of a different outcome in the longer term. There is much in life which could follow that template. If a trauma takes place in which nothing can be resolved at the time, it is important to lay down something that holds open a belief in the possibility of later enlightenment and resolution, and therefore a better situation.

In writing this book, I am aspiring to help to raise the awareness of any person who is responsible for a child to issues and imperatives that are often unseen or misperceived. The sense of true meaning that is inherent in the experience of real human connectedness is the very essence of life. Yet there is much that may interfere with the evolution of that connectedness between people. It is the awareness of such interference and its origins that allows us to strive to limit the impact of it.

We are all familiar with observing the physical development of a new person, right from birth. This development is enabled by the encouragement and validation of physical movement, and by encouraging and applauding the intake of adequate nourishment in the form of food and fluids.

However, nourishment of the growth of the emotional life and the psyche of each new person is not as easy to identify and describe. It is, of course, inextricably entwined with physical growth and development, but it is also a subject in its own right. The new person requires emotional nourishment in the form of ongoing specific, appropriate interactions with other human beings so that the emotions can be identified and validated in order to become 'installed'.

It is my hope and my intention that this book will help the reader to understand some of the central elements involved in the development of the emotional structure of human beings. I have attempted to explain in simple terms something of how such developmental needs present and can be recognised, and how they can be responded to and addressed appropriately.

This is relevant not only to the care of any child, but also to the understanding of unmet, and therefore unresolved, child-state needs within a person of adult years.

The stages of the basic human physical developmental process are universal. Delays and interruptions to this process can be provoked by physical interference or temporary damage. At worst, certain kinds of physical damage can halt the process, leaving the person unable to progress, or even causing death. Insufficiency of food or water can limit physical development, and prolonged absence of food and/or water can result in death.

The fundamental stages of the emotional development of humans, and what is required in order to achieve these, have been well documented and are universal. There is an almost unspoken expectation that the emotional nourishment which is required for each of these stages is provided by the birth parents, or those who are standing in place of them. But how do the parents acquire the knowledge and experience that is required in order to be able to provide that essential nourishment?

It seems to be assumed that parents, by virtue of their physical maturity, are not only capable of creating a new human being, but also can provide the emotional nourishment that is essential for the secure development of the emotional life and the psyche of their child. From where have the parents learned that art? It seems that no formal training is provided. Is this because it is assumed that no formal training is required? Should this really be the case for an endeavour that is so crucially important that the safety of the world depends upon it?

In the workplace, training is accepted as a central and necessary factor in the development of appropriate competence. For example, a boy who wants to become an electrician, and whose father is an electrician, may well learn a great deal about the subject by observing him at work and by listening to what he is saying. However, in order to become an electrician, that boy must undergo rigorous training – for the safety of society and of himself.

Each parent has been a child in the care of a parent. The emotional life of each person is the result of what he has experienced in relationship with his parents and other carers. Much of this has been absorbed rather than taught. Only a small proportion of that process is carried in the conscious mind. A child who receives adequate help with his emotions can later, as a parent, guide a child in the same kind of way, and this can take place quite spontaneously. However, if this is not the case, then a child in his care will at times receive inadequate or perhaps damaging interactional input from that parent. How is such a process monitored? It is largely the case that it is not. Only in the more extreme cases of difficulty may a child sometimes have a chance of receiving recognition of his inadequate or perilous situation, and also be given help for it.

For most people who do not receive adequate interactional input for sufficient development of their emotional life, the consequent gaps and insufficiencies limit their ability to interface with the world confidently and competently as they go through life. Some are quiet and withdrawn, some manufacture blustering behaviour or aggressive strategies in an attempt to cover up their emotional pain. At worst, emotional development can be arrested by severe emotional trauma. This might not be apparent if adequate physical nourishment continues. The physical body grows and matures, and this results in a person of adult appearance, albeit with emotional needs of a child.

For any person who is to be the carer of a child, it is well worth reflecting upon their own childhood experience of emotional nourishment, and to look at whether or not it was adequate. Was it limited in certain specific areas? Or perhaps interaction that should have been emotionally nourishing was instead actively damaging. Unless there is some conscious grasp of the significance of what each of us has received in this arena, there is a real risk that a parent or carer will merely replicate unhelpful patterns of interaction. These can be distressing to their child, and may risk limiting his development. The process of such reflection is one which ideally should be ongoing – to allow further review and consequent insight.

There are those who have never been in any doubt about the damaging effects of some of their childhood experiences. I believe that many of these people strive to ensure that no child suffers similarly while in their care.

Within the compass of this book, I provide some descriptions of certain kinds of interactions in order to illustrate for the reader relevant essential processes that take place in emotional development. I also provide examples of the consequences of inadequate emotional nourishment.

Each new person's need to develop emotionally is there,

waiting. His experiences with those who care for him will fulfil some of the elements of what is required. Gaps in this process, together with the presence of adverse input, can lay down patterns from which distortions can develop in the new person's inner state. Such distortions can lead not only to limitations in the way that that person interfaces with life, but also can manifest as physical distortion or pain.

Emotional security is the bedrock of a balanced life. It is the cornerstone of meaningful relationship, and of the experience of being part of the human race. Without it, real collaboration is impossible.

I am a therapist who has a detailed understanding and an extensive working knowledge of psychological processes. It is fundamental to my understanding of any person who comes to me for help that from the outset I elicit the answers to a number of relevant questions. For example, I need to know how many brothers and sisters were in the family, the order of their birth, and the age gaps between them. I need to know about their relationship with their parents – past and present – and I need to know what stressors were affecting those parents. I need to know if any of the grandparents, aunts, uncles, neighbours and friends were involved in their care to a significant degree. I need to know how many times the family moved home, when such moves took place, and under what circumstances. These are a few of the main questions that will begin to bring into focus for me the theatre in which the person in front of me did not receive sufficient help with his emotional development. The symptoms of stress, depression, anxiety, distress, panic, and so on, of which any sufferer might be aware, are a consequence of the presence or absence of events and interactional patterns which took place in that person's life experience – starting right from the beginning.

How can we prepare a child for life?

How can we prepare a child for life, when we do not know what the future might hold? Parents of children born at the end of the nineteenth century would have no idea that their offspring would have to face two world wars. And if they had known this, how could they have prepared them? The answers to such questions seem imponderable.

Parents of modern children know that they have brought new people into a world of rising sea levels, dangerous levels of pollution of the environment, and necessary focus on the 'carbon footprint', to name but a few common concerns. What must they do to prepare their children for adult life?

In recent times, during a visit to a large well-run primary school, the very experienced head teacher told me that although she did everything she could to prepare the pupils for their future, there were imponderable matters involved. She gave the simple example of handwriting. She explained that teaching children handwriting was still part of the central curriculum, but pointed out that more and more the use of computer keyboards was the most common way of writing. Could it be that in the future the skill of handwriting would no longer be needed?

As parents, we have to teach our children about day-to-day physical safety, and to help them to comprehend and observe the rules and norms of our current culture. However, the rules and norms of our society will change over time, and in a world where foreign travel is still prolific, many people will be required to observe and adapt to the rules and norms of cultures that are different from their own.

Changes within a culture can be confusing to the elderly, and they can be confusing even to those who are not yet elderly. At a hospital appointment some years ago, I was directed to lie on an examination couch. Having not been a hospital outpatient for some years, I was unaware of changes in protocols. I stood by the couch, and began to remove my shoes. 'Don't take your shoes off!' the doctor commanded. He did not seem angry or aggressive, but there was a force in his voice that I found confusing. Mutely, I secured my shoes, climbed on to the couch, and lay down, feeling frozen and a little tearful. Later examination of my feelings in the relative safety of being away from the hospital premises led me to consider how, as a child, it had been impressed upon me, very firmly indeed, that I must *never* climb on a bed with my shoes on. I had been left in no doubt that such an action would attract some kind of dire consequence – one which I had no desire to experience.

Although with the benefit of my adult awareness and intelligence I could imagine retrospectively that the doctor was acting on a need to limit the spread of infections such as MRSA, the child inside me was disturbed. In her early years she had been given an unequivocal rule about shoes, yet that had now just been completely countermanded, and without any warning.

This example led me to reflect yet again on the child's position. The first set of rules that are presented to him are, in his inner world, the *only* set of rules. How then do we prepare him for necessary change and evolution of the particular form of reality that has been described to him through such rules? How can we rear children who are intrinsically flexible? With the perils that our current world is presenting to us all, above everything else, we need people who are flexible, in a calm way. This is an essential prerequisite for the discovery and development of pathways that will help not only the individual, but also have the potential of helping every one of us.

Emotional security is the essential core of a balanced life. It is the cornerstone of meaningful relationship, and of the experience of being part of the human race. Without it, real collaboration is impossible. What we can aspire to do is to give our children the kind of interaction that they need in order to develop a secure internal emotional base from which to face the unknown.

In the beginning...

I was originally asked to write a book about childcare. In essence the subject is quite simple and straightforward, and yet the working through of it in the day-to-day living experience is so multifaceted that a single book could never aspire to address all its complexities. One could imagine that a book on childcare should have a coherent organised flow to its content. Yet by its very nature, the process of childcare demands an eternal flexibility.

The overall concept of childcare is really about the care that is required during the early years of life in order to enable the physical, emotional, and spiritual growth of a new person, and how an adequate amount of this care can be provided.

Adequate provision is fundamental. Readers might find Bruno Bettleheim's concept of the 'good enough' parent (a concept that is referred to by both D W Winnicott and by Bruno Bettleheim) to be helpful in the examination of what might be deemed to be 'adequate'. Some parents may long to provide 'perfect' care. If this is the case, I would ask that the concept of perfection is considered carefully. The world into which a new person is being invited is a complex and challenging entity, which is ever-changing. A parent can never hope to mediate every aspect of this interface perfectly, and it will gradually become plain that the parent has 'failed' in certain respects. Such 'failure' can be a consequence of factors such as inadequate factual knowledge, inadequate emotional development of the parent, lack of awareness that the child is experiencing a problem in the interface, and so on.

Truly adequate parenting must by its very nature include the capacity on the part of the parent to accept his or her current limitations, and a willingness to interact openly about this whenever needed. A mother or father who can say to the child 'I'm so sorry, I got that wrong. I didn't know it was like that. It would/might have been better if I had... Perhaps we could try again' is laying down a very important foundation. This foundation can help the child to develop an emotional tolerance of inconsistency, uncertainty and inadequacy, and to learn creative ways of clarifying difficult situations throughout his life.

If a child can experience inadequacy in a safe situation – i.e. a situation in which the wish to reach a 'better place' is demonstrated – he goes on to be able to mediate interactions with others confidently. Such a person has no worry that uncertainty and disagreement might provoke feelings such as anxiety or fear for him.

I think that a helpful approach would be to describe a series of situations – some fictional, and some real-life – and reflect on this material in a way that elucidates some of the 'unseen' aspects of the interactive processes that are involved. This is the purpose of the cameos – on pages 31-55. In this way I hope to raise the awareness of the reader not only to the needs of the child that requires the care in the here and now, but also to the needs of *the child of the past that dwells inside each 'adult' state*. This is of crucial importance, as it is not possible to provide care which is genuine and adequate unless the carer has, as a child, received a sufficient supply of such care *or has become conscious of the gaps in their own care and the consequences of such gaps*. A parent's or carer's acceptance of this situation means that the help that any sufferer of inadequate parenting gives to a child is far less likely to be contaminated with the 'adult's' need to attempt to conceal from himself any residual emotional pain from unresolved issues from his own childhood experience.

If a parent has had childhood experiences that have been

significantly painful, and that pain has never been adequately addressed, then it is not unlikely that the parent will give a less than adequate response to certain of the new child's range of needs.

Any parent would be well advised to be observant of the intensity of their own feeling states. Making a note of these, and the circumstances in which they occur, can help in the process of locating and understanding the origin of such states. It is commonplace, and all too easy, to attribute the whole of any such intensity to a particular situation that is presenting in the here and now. However, it is important to take time to reflect upon such assumptions.

Some of us might prefer to feel that because our own childhood took place long ago, it remains in the past, and has little or no significance now. Such a belief system is potentially very limiting, particularly if we have actual children in our care. Those readers who are familiar with Roald Dahl's book 'Matilda' will remember the Trunchbull making the loud declaration 'I was never a child!' It is obvious that her denial of her own child state resulted in her care of her pupils being of poor quality.

At this point I think that it is well worth writing something about the term 'temper tantrum'. The use of this, often angrily and disparagingly, saddens me greatly. When I hear it being employed I usually do my best to open out an understanding of what this state really is. In essence, it is a cry for validation of the feelings of anger and rage. Unfortunately, the state is often misinterpreted as the child being deliberately and wantonly 'bad' or 'difficult'.

The toddler, overwhelmed by a rush of very intense emotion inside himself, is often literally knocked over by the strength of it – falling to the ground, or throwing himself there, dominated by the internal disturbance, which he experiences as a driving force.

He has no capacity to modify this, and is taken over by it. He needs help. Instead he may receive hindrance in the form of being ordered to 'stop it' – or being told that he is naughty. Such hindrance serves to perpetuate the state in which the child finds himself, and his cries for validation of his feelings might well become more frequent and insistent.

What he needs is someone to be with him in his feelings of anger and rage – to name them, and to connect them with the situation in his life that has provoked them. The parent who can hold his child compassionately and firmly, naming the child's anger and rage, and acknowledging the fact that the rage might well be directed towards that parent, is well on the way to enabling this new human being to become an adult who is confident in relationship, who can use his feeling states appropriately and not be 'taken over' by them. He will be able to speak of feeling angry, rather than lashing out or behaving in other kinds of inappropriate ways.

For the parent who has not received compassionate help with the naming and validation of his own feeling states this is easier said than done – or merely 'pie in the sky'. Such a parent all too often finds himself in a situation where, faced with a 'temper tantrum' in a toddler, he will feel like shouting at him to shut up, smacking him, telling him that he is bad, or even shutting him in another room. A light shone into the early life of such a parent might well reveal that this is exactly what used to be done to him.

All parents are handing on to the next generation what they themselves received in their early years – when their baseline experience of life and relationship was laid down. The parent who as a child has suffered at the hands of ignorant 'parenting' is destined to exhibit hurtful 'knee-jerk' reactions to his own children that are based on what he had been exposed to, *unless* he understands and reviews the origins of his own pain. Conscious personal understanding of a sufferer's pain gives him an objective grasp of his situation, and provides the option of his reviewing his responses and actions, thus enabling him to be able to choose to behave sensitively and helpfully to his children – new human beings.

The plethora of so-called anger management courses currently available are filled with people who have not had the advantage of the kind of parenting that each child has a right to have – one in which their feeling states, whatever they are, are named and validated.

The difference between having a feeling state, and having one and *acting it out* is enormous. In an adult who is feeling murderous, the difference is pivotal to his life and to the life of the person upon whom the murderous feelings are focused. If the feelings are *acted out*, then both the sufferer and the victim are at serious risk – the former being at risk of being imprisoned for life, and the latter of losing his life. This might seem an extreme example to think about, but each of us, being human, has the capacity to feel murderous. It is not long ago in the history of man that personal survival depended at times on being able to act upon murderous impulses.

If murderous feelings are validated and truly understood, then the person who has them is not at risk of employing them in a driven way for the destruction of another.

A person who has not had his feeling states adequately validated in his early years is destined to be dominated by a need to have them validated now. He will present them in all kinds of ways in all kinds of situations, where they might look 'entirely plausible' or might appear out of place, both in form and intensity. His chances of having a particular feeling state validated at such times are very 'hit and miss', and his need for validation may re-present in various guises.

Some will try to cope by 'not having any feelings' – numbing them by internal effort, taking drugs (prescription or other) or drinking alcohol. This is the position of despair, where the sufferer of inadequate validation of feelings has simply given up hope that any other human will ever understand his need.

Some will insist, perhaps loudly and relentlessly, that their view on things is *the only one*. Some will become tearful, expressing misery that no one understands them. There are many other outcomes in which the sufferer becomes trapped, *unless the related early experiences are rediscovered, understood, and reviewed.*

The original deprivation will have been laid down in relation to another person. Addressing it in the present also requires relationship with another person – someone who understands the emotional mechanics of such dilemmas.

The demonstration of *true remorse* on the part of the parent is a crucial dynamic between parent and child. True remorse cannot be conveyed merely by saying 'sorry'. If that word is used on its own, it must be the embodiment of detailed and heartfelt awareness of the hurtful impact on the child of the actions of the parent.

In such situations, the parent may well need to make an appropriate distinction between the child's experience and the parent's original intention. This is a fundamental distinction to be able to make. In many of the stages of its early development, a child simply will not have the capacity to grasp the broader picture, and therefore might well not understand why the parent acted in a particular way at a particular time – albeit *in the best interests of the child.* All the child may understand is that he is hurting or angry about how the parent acted. In these cases, it is of central importance to validate the feeling states of the child *first.* Any attempt to explain to him that the parent was acting in his best interests either falls on barren ground or only serves to push a sensitive child into mute despair about his inner situation ever being addressed. This might become coupled with the risk of the child becoming someone who demonstrates more understanding of everyone else than of himself.

Being ready to communicate to a child, with unreserved genuine intent, that you can well see why he is feeling angry and upset, and to stay in this communication until certain that the child has absorbed this, and is feeling validated, is crucial. It is only then that the parent is truly free to explain more about the greater situation and his actual intentions for betterment of the child's position.

Here I have not made a distinction between needs at the different developmental phases. The same need is present in each. The only difference is that the parent must endeavour to speak at the level in which the child is best able to receive and understand.

I well remember a very long wait that I had to endure during a parents' evening at our son's secondary school. He had specifically asked me to see his percussion teacher, and although at the time I was suffering from severe sciatica, I was determined to fulfil this request. I sat on a table, I sat on a chair, I stood up, and I walked about. As always, nothing would relieve the pain. Each minute seemed like an hour. I longed to be able to go home and lie on the floor with my knees bent upwards, as this was the only way I could have some respite. But I had promised to see the percussion teacher, and stay I must. Then, at last, my turn came, and the teacher took me into the room where we would discuss my son's lessons. I cannot now remember exactly what I said, but I did burst out with something that was not entirely adult! The teacher looked straight at me, and apologised in an entirely genuine way. My emotional pain vanished and my physical pain became endurable. We talked about my son's musical gifts and skills.

It is not difficult to surmise from this that in my early life there were gaps in the validation process of my feeling states which had not been addressed since! I may well have been justified in feeling disgruntled about the long wait at the school, but the mode of conveying my feeling had not been completely adult.   As far as I can remember, the words I used were appropriate, but the expression on my face was less so.   The teacher's response had certainly reached deep into the core of my early deprivation, and I have valued this ever since.   He had offered something to me unreservedly, and *I had been able to accept it*.   I mention this because, in some cases, the person in my position might have blocked the human intention of the teacher, and might have gone on to represent dissatisfaction more intensely.   Such a person is not a 'worse' person than I.   He is someone who has a different set of inner problems with which to struggle.

Developing the skill of being able to perceive when we are manoeuvring with difficulty inside ourselves, and being able to operate within the varying levels and origins of difficulty, is challenge indeed.   Most of us have gaps in the kind of parenting we received.   How do we manage the impact of these, particularly in relation to our own children?   Justifying our behaviour, loudly and insistently, is likely to be a sign that we are failing to look more deeply and honestly at a situation.   Our children can be casualties of our failures to recognise and deal with our own emotional pain.

Some parents might, understandably, wish to have a manual to which they can refer with ease – about all 'practical' aspects of rearing a child.   I do touch on some of these.   However, any such considerations have to be set in the understanding of a much broader picture.

As a parent of three, and with a background in agriculture and nutrition, I could write much about food and feeding.   I could draw up tables of a standard healthy diet for different stages of childhood.   Adding a section about the diagnosis and management of food intolerances and allergies would be interesting, and would add more 'food for thought'.   A further section, about the impact on food quality of current agricultural and horticultural practices and also food manufacturing systems might enlighten the reader further. For example, would anyone want to risk feeding a child on a compote of pesticides that are commonly found in lettuces and carrots that have been grown without organic status? And yet even this breadth of examination would be incomplete.

Likewise, I could write about baskets, prams, cots and beds, their construction and suitability for infants and children, clothing and coverings for sleeping, how to keep a child warm, or cool, choice of sleeping place, and so on. But finishing there would mean that a central and absolutely crucial piece of understanding which is entirely relevant to the subject of sleep would not have been represented ...

The human embryo, developing inside its mother, relies entirely upon her for all the elements that it needs for physical growth. Deep inside her, it is protected. Throughout pregnancy, mother and child are one. The baby truly is *a part of the mother.*

At parturition, the single 'pregnant mother' form changes into a mother and a baby. The mother knows that this has happened. There is no doubt that the baby is no longer inside her body. This is a visible and palpable truth. However, the baby's situation is considerably different. The baby's experience is that he is still part of the mother. Not only is it logical for us to assume that to be the case, but also there is plenty of evidence which supports it.

Perhaps the single most important consideration in the process of growth and development of a new person is to take account of the inevitably slow and complex process of enabling that newborn person to discover that he is no longer part of the mother entity. In this slow evolutionary process, the child's discovery that he is no longer physically part of the mother is one that becomes apparent to him far sooner than the emotional and spiritual separation from her.

Daily, the baby will experience and re-experience the physical shock of separation from the mother's body. Slowly, very slowly, with help and compassionate understanding and handling, the baby begins to be able to experience himself as being attached to the mother *even when the mother is not holding him closely*, her breathing, heartbeat and emotions merging with his. Slowly, very slowly, with help and compassionate understanding and handling, the baby moves from the position of constant physical nourishment that takes place in the womb. Through this process, the baby is enabled to come to experience the sequence of separate feeding events that take place through the day and night as a *reliable feeding experience* – so that, although there are gaps between feeds, the overall experience is one of continuity. The sound of the mother's voice, the smell of her skin, and the mixing of these fundamental sensory stimuli with the baby's clothing, the material of the covers under which he sleeps and the aura of the domestic sounds around him begin to take the place of the womb experience as a safe situation. The infant experiences variations less and less as shocks or anxiety-provoking disruptions, instead accepting them more and more as the ebb and flow of mother's continuing presence in his world.

This process of the infant reaching an experiential understanding of his being a separate entity, in which he is cared for sufficiently, so that the separateness is no longer a shock, is a crucial step into embracing life. If we try to speed up this process, we run the risk of preventing a fundamental transition from taking place. Instead, we have an infant who appears visibly agitated, or who gradually learns to accommodate by no longer protesting about his distress. This latter state is fundamentally one of despair. (See the work of James and Joyce Robertson.) Such a state can form the beginning of the 'performing monkey' situation, where the child is prevented from expressing his natural impulses to be received and understood by the parents, and instead 'does what he is told', not understanding, and being diminished as a person.

I am not saying here that no parent should completely avoid insisting that a child behaves in a certain way. This in itself is an important component of survival. A child has to be told not to touch the flame of a fire. A child has to be told not to run into the road. A child has to be told not to eat certain beautiful berries that are poisonous. The key to the use of this kind of message is to deliver it with loving firmness. Only later will the child gradually develop an understanding of what burning, being run down by a car or being poisoned actually means. And of course it is not appropriate to force this understanding prematurely by deliberately exposing children to the consequences of such terrible events!

There are also very many everyday situations in which any child will need help to learn how to interface with his family, his peers and the whole of society.

* * * * *

The new person is waiting to be filled up with a sense of who he is. In essence, he is waiting to be filled up with himself. The new person is reliant on the people around him to reflect back to him the goodness in the substance of what he radiates. In this way the new person learns about himself and is slowly filled up with a sense of who and what he is.

Members of modern society do not have difficulty in understanding that a computer cannot do what the user wants unless relevant software has been installed. However, there are those who seem to think that children should be able to mature without any particular relevant input.

It should not be difficult for us to understand that unless a child is reared within a web of relevant interactions, he cannot learn about himself in a way that enables him to mature. A child needs ongoing appropriate interaction – based on facts and emotions – in order for emotional incarnation to take place. Appropriate interaction with parents and other caring adults leads to the child feeling confident and good about himself. Inappropriate interaction can leave the child feeling confused, and perhaps bad about himself.

It is important to remember that a young child cannot distinguish between an action being bad and a person being bad. The child can be left feeling that he is an entity of badness when in fact he has been told that what he had done was inadvisable, and should not be repeated.

If the new person learns about himself largely through an intelligent, kindly and compassionate interactive process, then he is instilled with a feeling of confidence. Helping a child not to do things that are deemed to be 'bad' is something that requires the use of a sensitive and intelligent approach that takes into account how the message will impact on the child's current capacity understand it.

Physical incarnation and 'emotional incarnation'

There is a profound difference between the process of physical incarnation and the process of emotional incarnation. The former begins at conception, and can be felt by the mother when the baby starts to kick inside the womb. The emotional incarnation is much more difficult to define. I often perceive it as a long, slow, process of interaction towards 'installation', the ongoing fine-tuning of which is essential.

Adequate interaction for emotional incarnation leads to the development of a strong sense of self in the new person – of who and what he is – whereas inadequate interaction, or damaging interaction, would lead to weakenedness and a sense of fragmentation. The body continues to grow, but the emotional structure has insufficient support and is vulnerable to stressors, leading to 'sagging' or fracture, which at times can be misdiagnosed as physical illness, or mental breakdown.

Early nourishment

When a baby is born, having only known life within a person, his perception is that he continues to dwell in a state where he is not a separate being. Any challenge that indicates that this is not so will fill him with intense alarm, and his normal reaction will be to scream as he feels torn away from what he can only perceive as himself. The baby needs a lot of close physical contact with a parent person while he discovers that he is not part of the mother any more. Developing a clear grasp of being in a separate body evolves over a period of many months, but the process of discovering emotional separateness takes far longer.

The baby has been born with a separate body, and daily experience gradually allows him to discover and perceive this. However, the perception and understanding of his emotions prior to his eventually being able to experience himself as a separate person is a process that is spread over years.

Feeding

Adequate feeding is essential for survival. A baby is born with a very strong instinct to suck, and this is for purposes of survival.

Instead of receiving continuous nourishment via the placenta, the newborn baby has to take milk into his body through his mouth. This taking in of milk is not a continuous process. It might feel to the mother as if it is continuous, as she will find that she has time for little else! However, the baby is in the process of undergoing a massive change, and needs small amounts of milk at frequent intervals while his stomach expands and his digestive system matures into the milk-dependent state.

If the baby does not receive sufficient milk, at frequent enough intervals, he screams – to alert the carer that his life is under threat.

As the baby grows, his stomach can take in more milk at any one feed, so that gaps between feeds become more apparent.

Although the taking in of milk is a vital aspect of the feeding experience, there are other crucial aspects that we must take into account. In itself, the process of sucking something is a nourishing experience for the infant. Not only does it mean that essential milk can be ingested, but also it means that a very deep need for reassurance about continued connection with the mother person is being met.

In addition to the provision of milk, it is not sufficient that only the need to suck is recognised and responded to by the parent person. Sucking is a very visible manifestation of a whole body need for contact and connection. Less visible are the requirements for the face around the mouth, including the cheeks, to be caressed, and the clothed body held closely. All this must carry with it a feeling of timelessness. Likewise, the whole body needs sufficient skin-to-skin contact, given in a loving way that carries with it a sense of 'forever'. Only then can the infant be reassured that life outside the womb is safe, and he can slowly move into a position where he can begin to experience short separations as part of a continuous process of closeness.

Loving eye-to-eye contact provides another fundamental channel of connection between mother and infant.

The infant does not only hear the voice of the parent through his ears. The head and body of the infant, held close to the parent's own body, absorb the vibrations of the parent's voice and body through his own. This is a deeply nourishing process, as it carries with it the resonance and reminder, and therefore the reassurance, of life in the womb. The vibrational quality of the parent's voice and its associated human intent – which form an entirely personal communication to the infant – are paramount.

In a calm and loving way the parent tells the infant what is happening around him and about life itself. Thus the parent nourishes the infant with goodness and sense. As time passes, the infant begins to respond by making sounds of his own that are the precursors of words, using facial expressions which are a part of his side of the 'conversation'.

Those people who in infancy have been denied sufficient sucking, skin contact and whole body contact are at high risk of smoking, overeating and other 'sucking related' activities, such as repetitive sexual actions, in their adolescent and adult years.

Sleep

It is generally recognised that sleep is a state which is essential for growth, restoration and healing. It is important that we do all that we can to enable our children to develop reliable patterns of sleeping. A child who is helped to experience sleep as an ordinary part of daily life is not only obtaining essential rest, but is also absorbing a pattern that will help him to be able to maintain healthy sleep habits throughout his life. Consequently this makes an important contribution to his ongoing wellbeing.

In the early months of life outside the womb, the baby is likely to be awake at night just as much as in the daytime. Frequent feeding is required, and the baby is kept close at hand at all times.

However, an external distinction between day and night can begin right from the start. Low lighting, low voice tones and a relative absence of playful stimuli help to define the night-time hours. The baby needs to know that the parent is still there – to demonstrate the continuation of the essential close link between them. This is the living out of the ongoing close connection that takes over from the constant nourishment and 'holding' that life in the womb provided, and is achieved by prompt response to the needs of feeding, close body contact, changing nappies, and so on.

It is not possible to prescribe a time by which a baby should be sleeping for longer periods during the night. This change depends upon a number of variable factors, and should never be forced. Eventually the time will come when the baby will sleep for much of the night.

When an infant is able to take in sufficient food through the course of the day to sustain him through the night-time hours, it becomes possible to define a 'bedtime'. Bedtime is the time when the parent will put the child in a cot, intending that the child will fall asleep and remain asleep throughout the night. Preparation for this separation is important and can carry with it very specific behaviour on the part of the parent which cues the child into readiness for a night's sleep. The parent needs to create a setting where the child has a strong ongoing sense of the parent's close continuing presence in his life, one that goes on all the time that he is asleep.

By the time the baby has advanced nutritionally to the point where he can sleep through the night, his recognition of being separate in a physical sense will have advanced, although this will not yet be complete. He needs ongoing fine-tuned help to discover that being a separate entity means that he is still strongly connected to another human, and does not mean that he is alone and abandoned, and cannot survive. He needs to experience physical separateness as a state in which his parent is *there for him* whether or not that parent is visible or palpable.

Bedtime routines for a young child often include the pleasure of playing in a warm bath of water, followed by being dried, and then dressed for the night – all of which allows plenty of time for prolonged close skin contact. A little more food, and quiet repeats of simple calm stories and songs, before being helped into the cot for the night with a favourite cuddly toy, are all things that can usefully be included. The parent might first cuddle the toy and the child together, very closely, kiss goodnight – in a lingering way – both the toy and the child, and continue to sing the quiet bedtime song when leaving the room and moving to a different part of the home. Some children might like to have a suitable soft object that belongs to the parent.

If there have been disturbing events for the child that day, it is important for the parent to take into account that some elements of the preparation for bedtime may well need to be extended in order to allow the child to enter the 'pre-sleep' state.

It is crucially important that the child hears a real human voice that is there specifically *for him*, and is *about him*. At bedtime, it might be tempting to leave the child to listen to a recording of a book or song instead of providing the essential personal input of one's own voice.

It is important to remember that to an adult person electronically-generated reminders of verbal and musical sounds are just that – reminders. They remind the person of what they have *already experienced and internalised*. Such reminders can never stand in place of real human sounds as a baseline experience of life. The vibrational quality is quite different. Any recorded 'reminder' can only be of positive relevance once the real experience has been internalised. The process of absorbing the real experience is complex and is multifaceted. It cannot and must not be rushed, particularly merely for the sake of 'convenience'. Impoverishment of baseline human experience is too high a price to pay.

Intellectual development

An infant who is well nourished both physically and emotionally can begin to look outwards into the world with an enquiring mind. He knows that he will be fed. He knows that he will have ongoing closeness with a parent. He is not agitated. He is not anxious about whether or not he will be given enough of what he needs. Certain of receiving enough, he can concentrate on and enjoy other things that come into his life. This is the earliest stage of intellectual development.

At several weeks of age, an infant can lie in his pram, watching the face of a glove puppet being moved slowly along the edge of the folded hood of the pram. He follows this face with his eyes, and tilts his head so that he can continue to see it. Then, expecting the face to appear on the other side of the hood, he turns his head swiftly in order to see it. An infant who is hungry for food and/or human warmth would show little or no interest in the puppet companion and its travels. He would be overwhelmed by inner signals for his basic needs to be met, and he would cry loudly.

A child who is taken to nursery or school without having been given breakfast, and without the ongoing knowledge of a warm reliable parenting presence in his life, is unlikely to be able to engage with much of what is provided in the way of intellectual nourishment. He may appear agitated, aggressive, 'clingy' or exhausted.

The child who is certain of an adequate presence of physical and emotional nourishment in his life is a child who is eager to reach outwards – to explore and examine, to seek and experiment.

Later on, it is possible for intellectual development to become out of balance with physical and emotional development. This can manifest in a variety of ways.

In a case where a child or young person shows particular intellectual aptitudes, that child may receive a preponderance of affirmation for these, with insufficient attention being paid to the need to validate other skills and aspects of his personality.

The footballer, George Best, seemed to me to be someone who must have received plentiful validation of his amazing skill in the use of a football. Sadly, it is quite likely that he received very little validation for anything else. Consequently his sense of himself depended almost entirely on playing football, and this put him at great risk of not being able to make sufficient sense of the rest of life – a situation which left him struggling.

It is very important that the maturation of the central personality is enabled to continue alongside the development of any particular gift or skill.

The young person who can write excellent essays and gain high marks in exams invariably receives much in the way of positive affirmation for this. But that person also needs to know that he is not being valued solely for this, otherwise his overall development can be out of balance, and there can be a risk that he becomes largely an 'intellectual performing machine'.

Re-presenting of feeling states

The importance of helping a young child to identify and name the feeling states that he experiences is paramount. This process is the bedrock of his becoming able to develop reliable and confident access to his emotional life, learning how to incorporate it into his interactions.

Once a child can name each emotion that presents itself inside him, he can communicate about them. For example, 'I'm angry.' Evolving on from there, he can form an approach such as 'Mummy, I'm angry with you.' And later, 'Mummy, I'm angry with you because you took my bricks away.'

At first, the big task of identifying and naming each emotional state is sufficient. Angry, sad, frightened, happy, worried... A child will encounter these states rising in a very physical way inside his body, and relies upon a trusted parent to help him with them. The naming of them is the first step. This is fundamental to all that follows in the development of his ability to use the knowledge of them in his interactions about events in his life that provoke such feeling states.

The ability to use knowledge of his feeling states in his communications enables the child to connect with and communicate about how events impact upon him.

A child's expression of happy feelings is likely to be received without any difficulty. However, in cases where events have provoked anger or sadness inside the child, a parent or other carer might struggle with this, particularly if they themselves are feeling distressed or are under some kind of pressure at the time. In such situations it is always possible to revisit the event later on, demonstrating an understanding of the child's attempt to communicate his feelings.

For traumatic situations where the child fails in his attempt to connect with the parent about his distress, the unmet feelings linger on, ready to re-present in a situation which brings them to the forefront once more. When confronted by a child who appears to be far more distressed by a situation than it seems to merit, the wise parent will begin to think about what else the child might be reacting to *at the same time as the obvious event*. It is important to attempt to identify the part of any big reaction that may well be a delayed reaction to an earlier event. The reaction may have been delayed by a failure to communicate about the significance of the earlier event, at the time or afterwards.

In the case of situations that are traumatic for the child and the parent, where understanding of attendant emotional states cannot take place at the time, the delay before these states are re-presented and recognised might span several years. During those years, it might seem almost as if the states do not exist. They have, in effect, gone underground.

The later turmoil of the adolescent state is one in which it is not uncommon to find signs of *something else being expressed as well*, and this can be something from early childhood. If not addressed at that stage, such states can reappear at other significant times in a person's life, such as connecting with a first boyfriend or girlfriend, or leaving home, making plans to live with a long-term partner or spouse, moving in together, having a baby, or when parents die.

Some cameos

When my first-born was small, I used to take him regularly to the big local museum, where there were all kinds of interesting things for him to see and do. He loved that place.

One day, I noticed a group of people standing together, each of whom appeared to have some kind of low-grade impairment. People who appeared to be carers were in close communication with them.

I was looking at an exhibit with my son, who was then about two years old, when there was a sudden sound of a very loud crashing thud close by. My son became quite agitated, and I tried to work out what had happened so that I could talk to him about it.

Through a growing crowd of people, I could see that one of the original group was lying on his back on the floor. He was wearing a kind of padded leather head-guard, and I realised it was likely that he had had an epileptic fit. I helped my son to get a glimpse of the sufferer as he lay there, telling him that the man had fallen over backwards. Then I moved away, explaining that it was important for us to let the carers have plenty of room to look after the man and help him.

I spoke to my son on many occasions about the man who had fallen over backwards in the museum, and how he had felt frightened, but that we had been able to see what had happened, and that there were plenty of people who were helping the man. And we told Daddy all about it when he came home from work that evening. However, any question of *why* the man had fallen over backwards had had to remain unanswered, as I could not think of a suitable way to explain it.

Before our son was one year old, my husband collapsed in the bathroom. Although our son hadn't seen him there, he had shown a lot of upset in response to the strange noises. A close friend, a neighbour, looked after him for an hour or so in her home so that I could attend to my husband.

When our son was a little older than three and his younger brother was about three months old, their father was in a car accident that had been due to icy road conditions. The car was a write-off. The top of my husband's head was bruised, and he was quite dazed. Apart from some other bruises, he seemed all right, considering the circumstances.

How could I explain to a three-year-old what had happened to Daddy, and where Daddy's car had gone? He hadn't asked any questions, but I knew that it was important that I helped him to understand something of what had taken place.

The next day, I took him on the bus, together with our baby in a carrycot, to where the car had been taken. When we found the compound, we peered through the fence and saw our white car, clearly damaged. He and I talked a lot about what had happened, and we told other people, too.

I felt very lucky indeed that my husband had not been seriously injured. The driving seat of the car next to ours in the yard had been squashed, so that the sides of it were nearly touching…

When our son was nearly four and his younger brother was nearly one, we went on holiday in the north of Scotland, and were staying in a wooden chalet in a lovely valley.

Early one morning, I heard a thud from the bathroom, and a distressed cry from my husband. I leapt out of bed and rushed to him, finding him on the floor, barely conscious, and retching. I covered him up to keep him warm, and made sure that he was lying on his side.

Later, he managed to crawl from the tiny bathroom into the living area, where our sons were now sitting, fully awake.

There was no telephone, and this was in the days before mobile phones. My husband lay on the floor, conscious, but very cold to the touch. Our one-year-old was crawling around him, patting him from time to time.

I waited for an hour, and at seven o'clock I went to the one neighbouring chalet and knocked on the door. The occupants kindly agreed to sit with my husband while I took my sons with me to the phone box, which was ten minutes' walk away. From there I phoned for a doctor, who was many miles down the valley.

The doctor came quite promptly and he radioed for an ambulance. Soon my husband was being driven away to hospital – a journey of forty miles.

How could I help my children? How could I explain to them what had happened, when I myself did not know? I told them that Daddy had gone to hospital and that I would get some news later that day. I knew that I would need money, so I planned to drive to the nearest bank, sixteen miles away.

At the bank a way was worked out for me to get some cash from our account. Feeling a little less vulnerable, I took the children to a phone box and rang the hospital. A nurse told me that my husband was 'just on his way to theatre'.

Then the four-year-old saw an ambulance parked just along the road, and he started running towards it. I had to help him to understand that Daddy was not in it, and I promised that the next day I would take him to see Daddy in the hospital.

That night, both the children were very disturbed. I accepted this as being entirely natural, and I lay awake all night in the double bed, with one of them tucked under each of my arms.

The next day I drove the forty miles to the hospital, and we found Daddy, lying in a bed, barely awake. I had to keep a close eye on our younger son, who headed straight for the catheter tube that was attached to the man in a neighbouring bed.

That evening, I did my best to pack all our things and clean the chalet, ready for an early departure the next morning. The drive home would take four hours.

Throughout the events that I have detailed above, I tried to do my best to keep in close communication with my children about what was happening. I had to work out what they could understand then, and what I must do to lay a foundation that could later be built on. Such a foundation would enable me to continue the slow process of helping them to understand and absorb the meaning of this challenge in their lives. There was no doubt that each event had caused emotional disturbance for both of them. In order to process this, they needed me to provide adequate communication about it. Such a platform would allow later examination and re-examination of what had happened, what people had done about it, and how everyone had been feeling. Many repeats, and the act of telling other people as well, slowly allow the experience to become meshed into the central understanding of the small person, at the same time enabling appropriate expression of the associated feeling states.

Should it be surprising that two particular girlfriends to whom our first-born later was drawn were people who suffered from medical conditions which could lead to sudden collapse? One was epileptic, and one was quite severely asthmatic. I did not intervene until there were signs that these relationships were foundering. At that point, when invited, I would try to help by making links between his troubled feelings about his girlfriend and the unresolved need from childhood to 'help Daddy'. When our son had been small, he had not been big enough to help Daddy, so that his desperate 'need to help' had lived on, and was now being focused on present-day sufferers of collapses.

* * * * *

When I am speaking to clients about the mechanisms surrounding the delayed expression of difficult feeling states, I usually begin by telling a story of a fictitious young child who has suffered the very ordinary experience of tripping and falling down, and has blood running from his knee. I tell this story to demonstrate what the normal sequence of events would be in respect of such a trauma to the child.

Not yet three years old, Toby is running along the pavement ahead of his mother, eager to reach the garden gate before her. She, wisely, is walking a little more slowly than usual, to ensure that he feels confident that he will succeed. Suddenly, Toby catches the toe of his shoe on the edge of a paving stone, and falls flat.

Poor Toby has no idea what has happened to him. All he knows is that he is in pain, and that he wants help from his mother.

Mother rushes up to him, picks him up and takes him home, saying, 'Oh darling, you caught your foot on something and fell down.'

Toby is sobbing loudly, but already he is being helped by the compassionate presence of his mother, who is explaining to him what had caused his world to become unrecognisable, and who he believes can help him.

Toby's mother keeps talking to him about what she saw happen to him. She has noticed that blood is running from his knee and down his leg.

'Darling, I can see that you've got a sore knee. When we get into the house I'll be able to help to make it better.' Actually, the mother is already starting the process of making it better, as she is helping Toby to grasp where some of the dreadful pain is coming from, thus confirming his reality in a helpful, containing way.

In the house, Toby may well first need some help with his hurt feelings. His pride at being able to move faster than Mummy has been destroyed, and has been replaced by a lot of pain. In fact, it might well feel to him as if *everything* is hurting badly.

Mummy wisely tells him how well he had been running, and what a lovely time they had been having (more confirmation of his reality). She goes on to say that he had had a shock when he fell over, and that she is going to help him.

The 'repair' includes the discovery of grazes on the palms of his hands, and exclamations of 'no wonder you're crying, that must hurt…' (more validation of Toby's reality) and so on. Validation of Toby's feelings must include the fundamental 'poor Toby, of course you're upset, you were having such a lovely time and then everything changed so suddenly.'

With adequate validation of the situation, the injuries, and the pain in his body and emotions, Toby may well not cry any more *even if he is still in physical pain*. The fact that his mother has demonstrated that she is *truly with him in the world of his suffering* has the power to make life feel okay again.

Further incorporation of the trauma and its meaning takes place in interaction with other people. When Daddy comes home, the whole story is told to him. When Auntie, Granny or a friend or neighbour calls round, the story is repeated. Kind, understanding responses serve to strengthen the link, endorsing, and adding to, what the mother had already established. Further sense is made of what to Toby had been the inexplicable destruction of his confident happiness by catastrophe. This cements his growing feelings of being okay again.

Such an event, together with competent handling of it, forms a wonderful template for any later trauma in a person's life. It has laid down the bedrock of the mechanics of an essential part of healthy human experience – one that brings sense and mending for the body and for the emotions – and forms an integral part of a trusting relationship that leads the new person confidently into life.

* * * * *

Many years ago, I noticed that a privately-run counselling organisation was advertising for therapists in my area to become part of their operation. I thought about this, expressed interest, completed the requisite application forms and sent them off. Some weeks later, I received a phone call from a woman who wanted to come and interview me. We made an appointment.

The interview was conducted in a semi-structured way, and this meant that I could bring into discussion relevant areas of mutual interest that perhaps no one had considered.

When the subject of family was mentioned, we exchanged some information about our children, and she confided that she was worried about her daughter, who was studying at college. Apparently, she had been involved in an accident where an object, dropped from a considerable height, had hit her head. Her recovery was not going as well as had been anticipated. I began to ask questions, including several about her daughter's emotional state and behaviour, and it became obvious to me that the recent accident was evoking memories of a previous trauma to her head, which from the finer details of the psychological impact, I realised must have taken place when she was an infant.

I explained this to my interviewer, whose demeanour changed immediately as she began to remember something that had taken place when her daughter was about one year old. She was visibly upset as she described this to me. She could see that the early event was directly relevant to the puzzle of how her daughter was behaving now.

For a few minutes I considered what to do next. This woman had come to interview me, and yet something of crucial importance to the understanding of her daughter's state was happening between us. I decided that the latter subject was the more important, and told the woman that if she wanted to, I could continue to discuss her daughter's situation, and that we could make another time to complete the interview. At this, she said that she would prefer to carry on with the interview, and I accepted that, believing that later she would put more thought into how to relate to her daughter's problems.

* * * * *

When I was first pregnant, my next-door neighbour was only a few weeks away from giving birth to her second child. She asked me if, when she went into labour, I would look after her first-born – a girl, aged three – while her husband took her to hospital. Although I did not know the child well, I agreed, as the only cover she needed was for the time it would take for her maternal grandmother to make the three-hour journey by bus, to provide the main source of help.

One afternoon, there was a knock at the door. The time had come, and the little girl was about to be brought round by her daddy. When she arrived, she appeared to be quite calm. She had brought toys with her, and she chatted to me in an ordinary kind of way.

Later, the time came by which Granny had been due to arrive, and I learned that the bus had been delayed. Mummy rang from the hospital, but the little girl declined to speak to her. Outwardly she still appeared to be calm.

Time passed, and there was still no sign of Granny… We continued with our playing and chatting.

Suddenly, the little girl screamed 'I want my mummy!' very loudly, and she began to sob. Instinctively, I knew that now, in her world, nothing else mattered at all. Any ideas of attempting to 'distract' her from her emotional pain did not enter my mind. I picked her up and sat her on my knee, wrapping my arms gently around her, saying 'Of course you want your Mummy. She is a lovely Mummy. Of course you want her.' This was the first stage of validating this child's sense of her current reality. To have her temporary carer agreeing with her that she wanted her mummy was central to her present need. I then went on to repeat everything that we had talked about before – that Mummy was in hospital having her baby brother or sister, and that Granny was sitting on the bus that was coming here so that they could be together while Mummy was not at home. This was another part of the child's reality that it was important for me to spell out as many times as was required, and so I did.

The cries and sobs and shouts continued, unabated, as one would expect. The only thing that mattered to this child was that she was consumed with a need to see her mummy, and she was expressing that very clearly.

I continued. 'You are telling me how upset you are that you can't see your lovely Mummy right now. *Of course* you are feeling upset.' I communicated this in genuine, heartfelt tones, thus conveying crucial validation of the feeling state that this child, by necessity, was having to endure.

It was fundamental that I should demonstrate sufficient understanding of her inner world, at the same time describing the relevant events in the world around her.

Eventually the child no longer needed to express her distress in the loud form any more. She sat quietly on my knee until Granny came, and then ran to her happily.

While they were still in my home, I told Granny, factually, that the little girl had been missing her mummy. The little girl had needed me, as her temporary carer, to connect with her granny (someone who was so closely aligned with Mummy, that she was a viable substitute) about her reality, and I could see by the girl's demeanour that now I had done so, she was content, and that life was fine again.

When my children were small, a friend of mine needed me to look after her two young sons, aged two and four years old, on a number of occasions. That family was under considerable stress at the time.

The younger of the two boys was behaving in a very disruptive way, disturbing or destroying the games of the other children, and he was unable to respond in an ordinary way to a range of the usual kind of creative approaches. It was obvious to me that he was full of angry distress, and that the only way he could express this was by making life difficult for his brother and my own children.

Eventually I picked him up and sat down, holding him firmly on my knee. As he wriggled and squirmed and fought me, I spoke to him about his emotions and his struggles. He was so angry that flecks of foam appeared at the corners of his mouth. Then he bit my arm. After this he was quieter, and was able to interact with the other children. He knew that I had understood his feelings and had accepted the expression of his rage.

* * * * *

Not long ago, my husband and I were away for a weekend in the Scottish Highlands. We had parked our car in a designated car park, just off the main road to Braemar. We went for a walk, and when we returned, a smart new car drew up quite near to ours.

A man got out of the driver's seat, and a woman and a girl emerged from the back of the car. This was clearly a father, a mother and their daughter, who was about three or four years old. I thought that although appearing to be following a Western lifestyle, they were of Indian extraction. The little girl looked beautiful. She was wearing a lovely dress, which came down to her ankles.

The man had a camera, and took some photographs of the scenery. Then he wanted his wife and daughter to pose together. The daughter would have none of this! She indicated to her mother in no uncertain terms that she was to step back, *well out of the picture.* The mother moved backwards a little, but this was not far enough for the satisfaction of the daughter, who insisted that she moved back further. Now content with the positioning, the little girl posed, smiling, for her father – several times. Each time the father took a photo, his daughter ran to check the screen on his camera to see if she felt happy with the image, before running back and waiting for the next photo to be taken.

The mother stepped forward to join her, but her daughter waved her away, angrily and emphatically. At this point, I worried a little about whether or not the mother would accept this. I knew that it was very important that she did, so I caught her eye, and smiled 'knowingly', trying to convey a message that she was reacting in entirely the right way. Thus engaged, the mother and I watched the next phase that was played out. The little girl moved to the front of the car, and did her best to spread the back of her body over the front of the bonnet, smiling intently at her father. I was sad that in our over-sexualisation of life this girl had taken in such images, but the innocence of her need to practise being 'Daddy's best girlfriend' was manifest.

Again, she checked the screen of his camera. Satisfied, she ran to her mother, pulled her into the area, and, snuggling up against her, ensured that Daddy took several photos of them together.

Watched by Mummy, the little girl had established that she herself was extremely attractive to Daddy – the most important man in her life. Safe in the context of Mummy's collaboration (and I believe, the mother's innate understanding of the developmental step that was being played out) she had insisted that she had a more important place than Mummy. Daddy had responded flawlessly to it all – apparently effortlessly, and entirely naturally.

I was so glad that I had been a witness (and possibly a temporary participant). I wished that such a scene could have been filmed and shown to all therapists and every parent to demonstrate this crucially important dynamic, which each child needs to play out in some form or another – the girl in relation to her father, and a boy in relation to his mother – in order to mature to the next step in the development of their sexuality.

Our current culture is full of people who are trapped with the need to act out what they could never express safely before. In the above example, if the girl had been prevented from doing what her natural impulses steered her to do, or worse still, had actively and deliberately been made to feel bad about what she wanted to do, then this could well have led to problems later on – first in adolescence, and if no favourable circumstances had come to her aid then, manifestation of problems could repeat at any time in the 'adult' years of life.

A failure to process a little girl's wish to express her need to be passionate about her daddy and be his best girlfriend, can result in that little girl, later concealed in the body of her womanhood, becoming fixated on the husband or partner of one of her best friends. Very sadly, this is not uncommon in our culture.

* * * * *

I was visiting a friend at the home of her mother, who was away at the time. My friend wanted to discuss some family issues.

When I arrived, my friend and her two-year-old son were playing with a railway set on the floor of the sitting room. I sat down close by, and she continued to play with him like this while talking to me.

Her son soon sensed that her mind was no longer primarily

upon the game that they shared. He tried to attract her attention directly, and, unsatisfied by her response and unable to focus on his game, he became irritable.

Not far from where I was sitting there was a small wooden stool. It had four legs, and looked very stable. On it was standing a tall vase. I had not taken much notice of this until…

The two-year-old, having decided that further steps were necessary to regain his mother's attention, looked intently at her. She did not notice the change in his demeanour. Staring at her meaningfully, he backed slowly in the direction of the vase. Once there, he stood next to it until she glanced across at him.

At that moment, he put one of his hands on one of the handles of the vase, and grinned at her. This had the desired result of his receiving focused attention from her.

'No! No!' she said in very firm tones.

Her son grinned even more widely, and shook the vase, his gaze never leaving her face.

There was more loud 'No! No!' from Mother, followed by a rugby-style tackle.

The vase did not get broken. It was clear throughout that the child had no intention of breaking it. He merely used the situation to ensure that he had his mother's full attention, and at that stage did not mind what kind of attention that was… His approach was entirely valid for his situation, and his age and stage of development.

* * * * *

It was a very windy day, and I had parked my car in a busy outdoor car park in town. I noticed that nearby a child aged about two years was standing next to his mother, and that he was clutching an open bag of crisps tightly. The mother was trying to encourage him to climb into his opened buggy, but he did not seem keen to do this.

Suddenly, the wind caught his bag of crisps and snatched it away from him, spilling its contents as it was tossed between the cars and out on to the busy road. The child was aghast. The mother told him that if he did not get into the buggy he would be blown away. She did not speak unkindly.

The horror on the child's face was manifest. To me it was clear that in his inner structure, he experienced himself like the bag of crisps, being torn away from everything he knew, and disappearing down the road. He grabbed desperately at the buggy, and climbed in, pressing himself hard into it.

I think that I have never evolved fully out of the position of a young child in respect of perceiving things quite literally. Although uncomfortable at times, this has been of use in my adult years in my roles as a parent and as a therapist. In fact, those years have made this capacity more apparent to me and have therefore allowed me to employ it effectively for good purpose. In many ways, it is of great value in my work as a 'detective' when examining emotional crises.

* * * * *

At the busy outpatient department of the local children's hospital, I was sitting in the waiting area with one of my young children. After a while, I became aware of a boy who must have been between three and four years old. He was wearing a heavy duffel coat, and as time passed, his face looked hotter and hotter.

I saw his mother trying to undo the toggles on his coat, but he would not let her. He grabbed the front of his coat, clutching at the toggles. She tried to reason with him about the heat, but he would not agree to take his coat off.

I puzzled about his reaction until I realised, with a lurch in my stomach about his predicament, that the last time this child had attended the hospital he must have been admitted as an inpatient. To him, taking off his coat signified that he would be staying in again. His mother did not press him, but at times tried gentle encouragement about removing his coat. He resisted, and she allowed this.

I said nothing, but sent from my heart a compassionate message towards him. I knew he would soon discover that after this appointment he would go home again, and that that would help him.

* * * * *

There was a boy aged four whose mother went into hospital. When she came home again, she had a baby with her. The expanded family settled into their new situation. Later, the boy's father had to go into hospital, and the boy was sure that when he came home he would bring a baby with him.

I felt uncomfortable when a psychologist gave this story as an example of failure in cognitive capacity. The cognitive capacity of the boy was well-developed and intact. As his only experience of hospital had been that a baby was brought home with the patient, he correctly assumed that this happened to everyone who went into hospital. On discovering that the next adult person to go into hospital did not come home with a baby, the boy was then in a position to review his previous assumption.

Of course, if the boy apparently had not noticed that a baby had come home with the mother from hospital, then there might well have been a cause for concern...

* * * * *

When Adam was an infant, he and his parents were living with his father's parents. In those days, a 'tin' bath being laid out in the kitchen was not uncommon. That household had this kind of arrangement.

One bathnight, Adam, aged one year, was under the kitchen

table. This was a position which was easy for him to adopt, as his head did not yet reach the underside of the table. The bath was to be filled in the usual way – with buckets of water. Just as someone passed the table carrying a bucket of scalding water, Adam ran out and collided with the bucket. He was badly burned and had to be taken to hospital, where he had to remain for nearly a week. This was in the days when parents could not stay with their children.

Adam has since had nightmares of starched white sheets, and the frequency of these nightmares is much increased if he has to attend hospital for any reason.

Adam was already emotionally vulnerable. His father's parents had some rather rigid views about life and about childcare, which they did not hesitate to impose in their home. In addition to this, there were signs that his mother had not bonded with him adequately. For example, family lore tells the tale of how she left him behind in his pram at the shops...

Throughout his life Adam has had particular difficulties in close relationships.

* * * * *

I was approaching a bus shelter on my way to the local shops when I became aware that a little girl there was clearly distressed. I saw that a woman was bending down to speak to her, and assumed that this was her mother, who would provide appropriate help.

As I passed, the child was crying and saying 'Ow! Ow! Ow!'

On my way back from the shops, I could still hear the sound of crying, and as I neared the bus shelter, I again heard 'Ow! Ow! Ow!' The woman grabbed the little girl and balanced her on the tilted metal shelf where people can be partially seated. Tears were pouring down the child's cheeks, and as she repeated

'Ow!' many times, she was pointing to her lower abdomen.

The woman appeared to be annoyed, and entirely unsympathetic. The girl's feelings seemed to be a mixture of distress and panic, and anger about what was happening to her.

To me, this child was in some kind of abdominal pain that she could not understand and therefore could not describe. I felt that if the woman could not manage to be kind to her, at least she could have asked a number of questions that would have helped to elucidate the problem.

'Is it hurting?' 'Show me where…' 'What sort of hurt is it?' 'Is it a needle hurt, or a bruise hurt or a very hard squeezy hurt?' 'Shall I rub it for you?' 'Shall I rub your back? That might help.'

I had a longing that the woman would show some real concern, but instead she continued to appear irritated about the situation. I was glad that the child was not silenced by this and continued to express her feelings authentically.

Having walked past, I combed my mind for anything I could do to improve things for that child. On balance, I felt that intervention from me, a stranger, could have made things worse, not better. The very important feature of the interaction between the child and the woman who appeared to be her mother was that the child *persisted* in showing her distress, and showed no hesitation or fear about doing so. In this respect, the child continued to manifest her reality.

I comforted myself with the knowledge that the children's hospital was only six miles away, and that if something serious was wrong with the child's health, medical help could be obtained quickly.

* * * * *

I heard of a little girl who was standing on a chair near the cooker, watching her mother making toffee.

The mother said to her, 'Now, don't put your finger in the pan because it's very hot, and will burn you.'

The girl was fascinated by the thick liquid in the pan, and longed for the toffee to be ready. As soon as the mother turned away for a moment, the girl put a finger carefully into the mixture. She did not cry out as she clutched her burnt finger.

When her mother saw her like this, she exclaimed, 'Oh dear! Have you hurt your finger? Let me see.' She then went on to help her daughter to look after her painful finger.

What would have happened if the mother had said, 'You stupid child! I told you not to put your finger in the pan. And don't come wailing to me. It's all your fault.'?

In this case the mother would have been venting her own disturbed feelings upon the child who needed her help. This would have been unlikely to improve the situation for herself or the child. The child had already learned that if she had followed her mother's instructions, her finger would not be hurting now. It was not necessary for the child's development or future safety to ram home a blameful message.

* * * * *

A child was walking along beside his mother in a shopping mall. He took from his pocket a small packet of sweets, the contents of which then spilled out on to the ground. I was glad to witness the following kindly response.

'Oh, darling!' exclaimed the mother. 'You've dropped all your sweets. Don't worry, Mummy will get you another packet. It's not all right to pick them up because they'll be dirty now.'

* * * * *

I once saw a substantial ancient vase in a museum. The vase was from around 500 BC. The pictures on it appeared in bands.

The top band showed several pictures of a newly wedded couple, gazing lovingly at one another. A change was shown in the middle bands, and the bottom one showed them glaring at each other. All signs of married bliss had disappeared.

I think that there must have been some unresolved material from childhood interfering with the interaction between husband and wife!

* * * * *

A television documentary about a nomadic desert tribe included tense scenes from a failing relationship between man and wife which were translated into English for the viewer. Apparently the husband had told his wife that she had a 'fat bum', and she was furious. She was determined to roll up her tent and go back to her family. A cousin of the husband came to attempt to mediate in this situation.

I was fascinated to learn that even under such harsh climatic and living conditions, such disputes were common enough. I don't know if the husband's boorish behaviour was due to endemic chauvinism, or whether it was because of bad parenting...

Another cameo: Boyhood and later life

In the days before antibiotics were discovered, it was common that a disease such as tuberculosis would cause the death of the sufferer. In the late 1800s, a certain casualty of TB was the father of a boy of nine. There were several children in the family, and this boy had an older brother, who then became the head of the family, even though he himself was only eleven.

The nine-year-old grew up and married, and in 1919, his wife gave birth to a son. He was anxiously watchful about the health of his son, and when that infant learned to walk, the father soon began to imagine that he was walking with a limp. He engaged the advice of medical professionals, and the only available treatment for TB was applied – immobilisation of the affected area. The tiny child was trapped, his pelvis in a plaster cast, and he was wheeled about on a kind of trolley arrangement. In nice weather the trolley would be pushed out into the garden and situated beside a flowering currant bush. His mother, and perhaps and aunt or two, would go to check that he was all right. He was well fed, was kept clean and was clothed appropriately, but no one connected with him about how he was feeling. No one sat with him and offered him comfort about not being able to move about.

This immobilisation lasted for nearly a year, and was later re-implemented, although for a shorter period. The son remembers how, when people came to him on his trolley, they would stay only long enough to serve his physical needs, and as soon as he showed any agitation or distress, they would rush off, busily.

After his final release from the plaster, the specialist in charge declared that she thought he had not suffered from TB at all. But by then a pattern had been embedded in his emotional structure. This was that if he were trapped, the people upon whom he depended would ensure that he remained so, and that if he showed distress, those people would leave him, to attend to something else, as if it were more important than he.

The child grew up to be strong and active. However, fearing that his son had been weakened by the 'illness', his father did his best to limit his activities. For example, when the son went to secondary school, his father arranged that he should not engage in sport.

After he left home, he spent time abroad in the army during the Second World War, and thereafter loved walking and rock climbing in the Scottish Highlands. He remained active throughout his seventies, and was still accomplishing lengthy walks in his eighties.

The time came when he was not so strong, and one of his legs manifested a neurological disturbance, which resulted in an intermittent partial collapse of its function. He could no longer do much of what he had previously enjoyed. He did not like this at all.

Things finally came to a head one November, when viciously cold weather had come early, and pavements were covered in packed snow, much of which turned to ice. The fracture clinic at the local hospital was flooded with patients, and although the orthopaedic operating theatres were working day and night, they could not keep up with the essential work of pinning and plating the shattered bones of the wave of casualties, young and old.

Now ninety-one years old, he slipped on a patch of ice just outside the sheltered housing scheme where he lived, and fell heavily on his dominant arm. He was helped up, but when he reached his flat, he found that his arm would not make its usual movements, and he phoned for help. At the local A&E

department, an x-ray showed a fracture at his elbow – in the upper part of his ulna – and one at the upper end of his humerus.

Most of his arm was then *put in plaster*... This put severe limitation upon what he could do for himself, and moving around became very difficult. It was clear that he would not be able to manage at home in his flat, and a bed was found for him on a suitable ward in the hospital.

A few days later, the man in the bed next to him developed severe diarrhoea, and soon after that the other men in the room fell ill, too. Norovirus was on the rampage through the whole ward, and people were asked not to visit.

Destabilised by his broken arm, and greatly weakened by the norovirus, he fell on the floor and could not get up. He was helped to his feet and back to his chair. He was told that he must not attempt to walk about on his own, and because members of staff were so busy, this meant that he spent most of the daytime hours sitting in a chair, unable to see out of the high windows. Thus he was in a situation that was not dissimilar to that of long ago, when as a tiny child he had been trapped and immobilised in a plaster cast.

A further complication was that during some nights his mind would revisit, as if in the here and now, the army hospital where he had been nursed with dengue fever nearly seventy years before.

Several weeks later he was transferred to a rehabilitation hospital, where he shared a ward with seven other men. This ward was spacious and airy, with plenty of daylight, and trees could be seen through the windows. Still he could not move from his chair without help. Because his formative experience of being encased in plaster was one where not enough of the help he needed was provided, he found himself completely unable to ask staff to help him to get out of the chair and move about.

Later, when a physiotherapist came to see him, he learned to walk with a zimmer frame, but he was very anxious about moving around unattended, and he found what seemed to him to be a vast expanse of floor in the middle of the ward to be too daunting.

Gradually he became a little more mobile, and then eventually the plaster cast was removed from his arm. Now he began the long process of working to straighten out the bent limb, and strengthen its wasted muscles. The hospital discharged him back to his home.

He had been heavily dependent on others for nearly eight weeks, and his current dependent needs were still considerable. Back home in his flat, care workers came in four times a day. He did not like this. *He would glare at them angrily, having to endure the minutes until they went away.*

It was very clear that the hurried visits of the care workers provided a context in which he suffered the same feelings as he had suffered as a small child, trapped in a plaster cast, without emotional support. Now he was trapped in his flat, with limited mobility, and until very recently had been immobilised because of his broken arm that was covered in a plaster cast.

He used to say that the people would come in and do things for him, but did not want to relate to him as a person, and would 'rush off' as soon as they could. The 'rushing off' element of the visits was deeply significant to him. Of course, there was a truth in his perception of the rushing, as these people had to visit several other homes within a set period of time. However, as the overall situation was so closely aligned to that he had had to endure as a small child, he was convinced that they did not care about him as a person.

In a desperate attempt to shield himself from the unresolved painful feelings of the past that were attaching to the circumstances of his present-day care plan, he tried to convince everyone that he did not need the care workers to come. His inner struggle was as follows. If they did not come, then he would not have to watch them going away, and the feelings of torment from his early life that he was having to suffer in relation to seeing the present-day departing person appearing to rush off would not have to be endured.

Deeply entrenched in the feelings that had been generated by the adverse events in his young life, and having insufficient in his present life that he perceived to be different from his early immobilisation, he struggled on. All attempts to discuss his emotional struggles with him did not get through to the problem at that time.

Little by little he was able to do more for himself, and it was not until this process was quite advanced that he could understand the sensitive sympathetic interpretation of his behaviour and attitudes of recent months.

Eventually, accompanied by a carer, he was able to walk along the street with the aid of a three-wheeled walking frame. Out in the open air, he discovered the way back to feeling himself again – the person who was no longer trapped.

Any later illnesses that led to long periods of time when he was unable to go out and about would lead to further revisiting of the painful emotional states that had been laid down during the entrapment of his early life, but his capacity to understand them was less fragile. Gradually, he became more consciously aware of the anger and frustration that he had felt as a small child when he had been immobilised. Although still very painful, these feelings became less likely to overwhelm him, and his tendency to feel despairing or emotionally frozen became far less pronounced. In fact, he began to view such states with some objectivity, laughing about the times when he still glanced at care workers out of the corner of his eye, with a dark expression on his face.

If, when he was trapped in a plaster cast as a small child, someone had been alongside him, giving him emotional warmth, understanding his feelings and validating the authenticity of these feelings, his emotional experience of later immobilisations would have been considerably different.

The pre-ruth state

The understanding of the pre-ruth stage of development is of fundamental importance in the care of small children. In the earliest years of development, the infant or toddler has no concept of how his actions impact upon those around him. He cannot take into account the effect, upon another person, of acting out his impulses. He has no awareness of the direct links between the acting out of his impulses and their impact upon another person. Such is the pre-ruth state.

The ability to exhibit ruth-less behaviour can only develop once the pre-ruth stage has been completed. A child who, because of appropriate help and guidance, has come to understand that his aggressive impulses, when enacted, can cause hurt or harm to another person, is in a position where he can *choose* whether or not to hurt someone. If he goes ahead with causing hurt or harm, then he is exhibiting a certain degree of ruthlessness. The enactment of ruthless behaviour requires its own kind of help from parents and carers.

It is common for a toddler to bite when driven by an aggressive impulse. If, when a carer or companion is bitten, that person shouts 'Ow!' and his or her face distorts, the toddler is likely to react to this by laughing. The noise and the funny face are amusing, in the same way as if someone were jumping around cheerfully while singing a silly song. In the pre-ruth state, the toddler has no awareness that there is a link between his biting and the expression of pain by the one who has been bitten.

How can we help the toddler to make the crucial link between the acting out of his aggression and the consequent suffering of another person? And, once that link is made, how do we help him to understand the consequence of his actions upon another? How do we help him to mediate his aggressive instincts in a way that initiates productive interaction? This whole process requires much patience and ingenuity, and is spread over a considerable span of time.

Making the connection for a toddler between his act of biting me and the appearance of toothmarks in my flesh will include repeats of a slow gentle demonstration of what happened. In a similar way I would help him to grasp that the bite had caused me pain, and I might engage him in 'helping to make it better'. Such understanding is the foundation from which one can insist that the toddler does not attack another child, thus avoiding hurt or harm.

The reader might be interested to know where my own developmental process has left me. I was recently queuing in a large airport with my small wheely-case. When I encountered an obstruction to its smooth progress, I pushed a little harder, and found to my horror that I had hurt the back of a young woman's foot. I was completely mortified. I didn't know what language she spoke, so I mimed my abject apology as best I could. She reassured me that it was okay, and that this kind of thing happened quite often. There could have been no doubt in her mind that I had not intended to hurt her in any way at all, and that I was *feeling with her the pain that I had inflicted upon her*. This is a good example of the expression of true remorse – an essential part of any genuine apology. My behaviour certainly did not stem from the pre-ruth stage, and it was not ruth-less – i.e. it was not carried out with the intention of hurting or harming.

The pre-ruth child does not know that he has hurt someone. He may see that someone has been hurt, but he has no idea that it is he who has caused the harm. To him, his aggressive act and his awareness of harm having taking place are two entirely separate states.

If the infant is not enabled to evolve from the pre-ruth position, the worst possible outcome is a person of full adult size and years who is unaware of the adverse impacts of what he is doing. Such a person can create mayhem in society – a psychopath.

This is quite different from the person who knows how his behaviour is likely to impact upon another, but deliberately goes ahead, knowing that the other will be hurt or harmed. He either wants that to happen, or is consciously uncaring about any damage caused. Such people are ruth-less.

And how is a ruthless person created? Having picked up that his aggressive actions impact adversely upon others, a child who is being exposed to damaging interactions – with or around him – can then go on to use aggression for the specific intention of dominating other people in order to get what he wants.

My daughter and I were sitting in the very large waiting hall of an airport, on a row of seats that were back-to-back with another row. We became aware of a man directly behind us who was using his mobile phone to speak to someone in an undisclosed location.

'Go and break his legs,' he instructed.

I think that there must have been some resistance from the person to whom he was speaking, because he then insisted:

'He [did something I didn't like], so *go and break his legs!*'

We froze. Was this some kind of spoof, or were we sitting back-to-back with an entirely ruthless person, who, when annoyed by someone, had ordered the destruction of that person's ability to walk? A terrifying prospect...

Then we were called to our departure gate. But the memory of that experience has stayed with me, lingering on in my mind.

An angry three-year-old, enraged by the behaviour of someone around him, can lash out at an adult, but do little or no harm because of the difference in body size. A parent or other carer must help the child with his angry feelings.

Where two young children are grabbing the same toy, and are

about to come to blows over it, the parent or carer can suggest and enable situations where a toy is shared. Perhaps the toy can be used first by one child and then by the other. Some other, similar, toy can be introduced, and so on. If all fails, the carer can, firmly and kindly, decide that 'the best thing is to put the toy away for now'. There are many constructive approaches, none of which might be perfect, but most are helpful in the long process of aiding the personal and social development of children.

In recent times, I encountered a seventy-year-old man who, although at first seemed pleasant and collaborative, actually dwelled in a state in which the only thing that really mattered was to get whatever he had decided that he wanted.

This became clear when he and I disagreed about something. Having failed to coerce me into adopting his view, he then quickly switched to the use of lying, verbal aggression and taunting, specifically with the intention of dominating me. His 'plans' of how things could be resolved were based entirely on how I – the unfortunate person on whom he had focused his rage – should cave in and 'behave properly', i.e. grovel and serve his loud demands.

When he realised that this approach was not bringing about the effect that he wanted, he informed me that he would blacken my name to a number of local people. It was clear that he intended to use further lies to achieve this end, and that he wanted to ensure that I would suffer isolation and misery because of his actions. There was no doubt that he would carry out this threat, determinedly and entirely ruthlessly.

I soon realised that this person was enacting what he had experienced as a child at the hands of an angry parent, but this time *he* was the 'powerful parent', and he had cast me in the role of the *bad child*, who had no power to avoid this 'awful fate'.

Having observed that any attempt at discussion or negotiation about the present-day issue resulted in his shouting louder and not taking account of anything at all of the relevant things I was saying, I ceased to attempt to talk to him. Internally, he was trapped by a pattern of interaction that had taken place decades earlier and had continued throughout his life. A friendly note from me resulted in his producing a badly-written tirade of vituperative ravings. I then knew that something fundamental would have to change before he could hear, and take in, what I was saying.

Of course, I wished that none of this had been the case. All I wanted was some kind of collaboration and mutual respect, but at the time this was not possible.

Clients come to me for the specific purpose of attempting to elucidate and modify problematic interactions in their lives. It is not uncommon for a client to disbelieve or struggle against what I am saying. In fact, this is usually a necessary part of the process. However, the context in which we meet includes an agreement to reach deeper understandings, for the benefit of the client.

The man about whom I wrote above could not admit that there was anything about himself that he needed to talk about. He was consumed with rage and with his determination to make me suffer. He is a person who might phone the police to complain about the behaviour of people who do not fit in with his decisions of how things should be. His complaint would be a deliberate distortion of the truth. He would not want to admit that his tales were flawed. The little I have learned from others about his father's behaviour towards him when he was young is sufficient to explain the origins of his behaviour, but it cannot help in the process of direct relationship with him. A pattern of relationship in his early life had left him with a drive to hate someone, and for him to be right all the time, and I have been a focus for his hatred. I have known others who, before me, have been placed in that uninvited role. I expect that at some time in the future someone else will become the focus instead of me.

Modelling

In the animal and bird kingdoms, unless the young follow and copy a parent, they are unlikely to survive. Consequently it is not surprising that the instinct to follow and copy is very strong.

In the case of humans, that instinct is present, and for the same reasons. One therefore expects that the young will copy a parent. This copying takes place not only when the parent is encouraging the child to copy, but also when the parent *is not aware that the child is observing and copying.* Not only does the child mimic a parent's actions, but also the child drinks in the very essence of who the parent is.

The parents may well decide to choose to exhibit certain behaviour and belief patterns around their children, in an attempt to impart certain attitudes. This is a creditable exercise, and one which I am sure frequently bears fruit of a positive nature. However, the parent must remember that it is not just the lessons that they consciously intend to convey that affect the child. The child absorbs *everything* about the parent.

As the child grows and develops, a female child will model herself primarily upon the mother and a male child upon the father. After all, these people are not only the people who created the child, but also they are representatives of male and female roles in the society into which the child has been born.

Some simple examples of modelling:

My friend and I had agreed to meet in a local café, where there were high chairs for small children. Her son was then about nine months old.

When I arrived, my friend and her son were comfortably installed, and she stood up to greet me. Being taller than I, she leaned forward, affectionately placing the side of her head next to mine. Her son was watching us intently, and I saw that as he observed us he moved his head in exactly the same affectionate gesture as his mother.

A friend with her two-year-old son had been to see me, and they were about to leave. The little boy was placed in his car seat, and the mother was putting her bag in the back of the car. The boy turned to me, and clearly had something important to say. I waited while he searched for the words. Then he said, in mature tone and verbal expression, 'I hope that you will come and visit us soon.'

In the local supermarket, I noticed a mother was standing talking to a man who was promoting a household product. Her two children – a girl about seven and a boy about four – were standing with her. The mother and the man were engaged in what turned out to be quite a lengthy discussion. I became aware that the girl was watching this intently.

While her mother was speaking, the girl watched her face and listened carefully. In between, she checked the input of the man. When the mother concluded the discussion, the girl, modelling herself on her mother, confidently added something similar of her own.

When, as a young adult, I left home, I was in a situation where for the first time I was doing all my own cooking. In those days, vegetables were seasonal commodities. Autumn came, and sprouts became available. Although sprouts were a vegetable that I had not prepared before, I found myself handling and cutting them in a very particular way. It dawned on me quite quickly that

I was unconsciously replicating exactly what I had seen my mother do.

Some possible complications:

If the parent is consistent in his or her behaviour, the child's position is likely to be relatively straightforward. However, if the parent's behaviour is significantly inconsistent, and this inconsistency is never referred to or explained, then the child can be left with a substantial level of inner conflict and confusion. In that way, the child can be exposed to two kinds of mummy or daddy, but within the same person. Switching from the task of modelling on one kind of mummy, then on the other, then back again can be confusing and exhausting, leaving little energy for the development of creative skills.

A very stark example of difficulty for a child can be found where a parent has committed a serious crime. If the father of a male child has been convicted of murder, how does the boy manage his survival instinct of copying his father, his male role model? In essence, the boy needs to be free to ask his mother (or other significant adult), 'When I grow up, do I have to kill someone like Daddy did?' It is unlikely to be sufficient to tell the boy not to be silly, adding 'Of course you don't' or saying something worse such as 'If you do something like that, I'll never speak to you again.' The boy is likely to require a discussion which includes the valuing of positive aspects of his father's personality, while confirming that Daddy had done something that was very wrong – something that no one should ever do.

The presence of a range of significant adults in a child's life is a factor that can modify the impact of any problematic behaviour of a parent or limitations in a parent's personality. The child can observe alternative forms of approach in the other adults, and may learn to discern the value of these alongside what he receives from a parent. His ability to see different approaches is enhanced if someone significant is able to discuss the fact that differences are present – thus enabling a child to develop a conscious grasp of similarities and differences. This is the beginning of the development of objectivity.

Two anecdotes:

Our daughter, aged nine and very familiar with our acceptance of feeling states, was deeply offended when Grandad told her that she couldn't be angry in his house, and that if she wouldn't stop it she would have to go out into the street. She rang me to tell me about this, and it was clear that to her, Grandad was *wrong*. Conversely, if she had grown up with Grandad as her father, and had been visiting us, she might have been surprised by the situation regarding the ordinary expression of angry feelings in our home. Further, if we had had conversations about how in some households the expression of angry feelings was not allowed, she may well have thought to herself 'Oh, Grandad's house must be one of the places where people don't show it when they are angry.' I think that her feeling of outrage must have stemmed from the fact that in her mind Grandad was an integral part of our household, as he had stayed with us many times. So it must have been that to her Grandad was being *wrong* and *bad* by putting an embargo on her angry feelings, rather than that Grandad was just a bit different in some ways when he was in his own home. From my point of view, of course I would have preferred that Grandad had not tried to crush the expression of her angry feelings. Yet I knew that however hard he tried, he would not be able to extinguish who our daughter was in the sense of her knowledge of herself, angry feelings included, that she had already developed in interaction with us.

When my father died, my mother came to stay with us for a month. She was in bed nearly all of the time, but as the bedroom was downstairs, she was part of family life. One of our sons, then aged four, was not able to form quite a number of his words correctly, and she did not like this. She was unpleasantly forceful in her insistence that he spoke properly. I found this situation difficult, as I believed that he would surely experience her approach as hurtful, and I looked for ways of protecting him from this. Our son assures me that he liked Granny a lot, except for the time that she disturbed one of his garden games in favour of the birds. I can only surmise that because our immediate household was one in which his way of speaking was not attacked, he relied upon that baseline experience and was not prey to being adversely affected by Granny's unkind attitudes.

It is well worth repeating:

Infants and children constantly copy what they see happening around them – *particularly the behaviour of the parents and other significant carers.* Many parents will discuss with one another certain precise messages and behaviour patterns that they wish their child to take in and replicate. This can be a very creditable and useful approach in a wide range of situations, but one has to be everlastingly aware that potentially the child is taking in *everything* that the parent does and says, and not just the aspects that the parent consciously rehearses and presents.

A word about some other influences...

What about the television screen that takes up a prominent position in the living room of many homes? How will an infant or a small child experience it? The screen itself is inanimate and mute, but when it displays programme material, it is the opposite of that. The images and the sounds that accompany the programmes are largely devised to attract and hold the attention of potential viewers, and children are vulnerable to this. Infants and young children do not have the capacity to apply objective reasoning to what they see. To them, whatever appears on the screen and whatever sound track accompanies this is *an integral part of family life.*

The question of whether or not such influences should be a part of family life is one which has undergone extensive debate, and no doubt this will continue. The plain facts are that infants and young children absorb *wholesale* what is going on immediately around them. They do not have the capacity to filter the material or apply an objective overview. The impact can be modified by the presence of a discerning parent who selects viewing material carefully, and who talks to the child about any material that is being viewed – thus making it a part of an *ongoing, real, meaningful, human relationship.* Without this, there is a risk that the child absorbs the material as if it were part of the family life of the household, and as if the people seen on the screen were the equivalent of extra family members.

How much do we want our children to model themselves upon what they see on a screen in the living room?

As television programmes are part of our social culture, it is important that we enable our children to learn how to live alongside them and in relation to them. This is different from wholesale, unmodified exposure to them. The latter state risks our young offspring taking in certain value systems that are not in their best interests.

It is inevitable that children will observe their parents' usage of mobile phones and other such items. It saddens me greatly to see a parent walking along the street, mobile phone clamped to an ear with one hand, the other hand guiding a buggy containing a child

66

who is being ignored. How can a child possibly comprehend the implications of Mummy appearing to prefer a lump of technology to the importance of her relationship with him? In truth, nothing can surpass the wonders of interaction with a developing human being whom she created, yet she hungrily devours sounds from the appliance.

Is it any surprise that children 'want a mobile phone' at a younger and younger age? They are modelling themselves on their parents' behaviour, and, most importantly, they want the feeling of connection that the parents apparently display in relation to the lump of technology. What these small children actually want and need is real human closeness and connection, directly applied to themselves.

I would ask the reader to consider the possibility that parents who spend much time attached to mobile phones may themselves be seeking something that plugs the gaps in their baseline feeling of connection to their own parents.

Would you want your child to be more profoundly connected to a television screen or a mobile phone than he is to you? Would you wish a new human being to perceive inanimate objects as being more significant than the other humans around him? Here we have elements of traits that appear in the so-called 'autistic spectrum disorders'.

The sense of agitation and inner disturbance that a child feels in the absence of secure connection with parents or parent figures is often displayed quite overtly. Such displays are not always easily definable as being different from conditions such as attention deficit disorder.

I am sure that any discerning parent would be able to extrapolate from my comments about such influences, applying careful thought to the situation of televisions in bedrooms, and to the use of computers for young children. However, in an era and a culture where the use of a wide variety of 'screens' is so very prevalent it is crucial to reflect upon the impact of such exposure on our children. Exactly what is a child absorbing from the 'screen' material? And what happens to a child who is in the presence of a parent whose attention is apparently fixated on a screen?

Even material that is promoted as having been devised for educational purposes should not necessarily be accepted as being suitable for young children to view. Do you want your child to be able to mimic and parrot material that has no real depth to it, or do you want your child to be encouraged to think creatively and develop independent thought? Do you want your child to learn from real human beings, or from flashing images of those who purport to educate or 'entertain'? How can we ensure that our children's predominant experience of life is formed in a context of genuine direct human interaction? These are some of the many questions that might help us to clarify our views.

'Screens' require that we use our vision in 'fixed focus'. This is true of any viewing, whether it is of close-up people or of a scene that includes distant mountains. The eyes are trapped in a fixed focus even when being presented with an illusion of variation. Without actual variation in focus, the flexibility of vision – 'accommodation' – can become limited. I understand that more and more children are becoming afflicted by this condition. With appropriate eye exercises and perseverance this can be reversed, so that a child's range of vision can be restored, but why allow it to become limited in the first place?

It is not uncommon for children and their carers to stare at a screen for long periods of time, blinking only rarely. Blinking is an essential part of maintaining eye health. Not enough blinking can lead to drying of the surface of the eyes, causing irritation.

A child who has a secure sense of connection with his parents explores what is around him, safe in the knowledge that someone is alongside him in his discoveries. A child cannot interface safely with a container of weedkiller, so a parent would keep such items out of reach. A child can be taught how to use a pair of scissors safely. Scissors are potentially dangerous, but with adequate supervision and comprehension a child can discover and enjoy the benefits of employing them creatively. Supervised access to watching certain carefully selected material that is portrayed on a screen may provide scenes that are of interest to a child and his parent, but this can never replace direct interaction between the child and a parent about the subject matter.

Separation

At first, Mother, or the mother person, is experienced by the infant as an extension of himself. Created by two people, the embryo inside the mother develops into a foetus and then a baby. The baby can only experience itself as *an integral part of one entity* – the mother's body. This cannot change during labour, or at the moment when the baby is born, as he enters the world outside his mother. The baby's experience is that he is still part of the mother. (See pages 17-18.)

The mother person is there for the baby in a very particular capacity. The baby does not know, and cannot know, the full extent of who the mother actually is. This is only something that is discovered later, over a long period of time.

As the child, later a young person, gradually evolves and develops, he slowly becomes less and less dependent on the mother person, both physically and emotionally. This slow progression eventually creates the setting in which the new person can begin to discover that his mother has a personality of her own, rather than his continuing to perceive her wholly and solely as an anchor for him.

An essential part of the process of the new person separating out into an individual in his own right depends upon his being able to develop the capacity to see in a broad sense who his parents really are as people. A crucial aspect of the enabling of this process is the parents' ability to engage in a way that defines and respects similarities and differences between them and their child.

It is imperative that a child models himself upon his parents in a variety of fundamental ways. However, there will be aspects of his perceptions, interests, attributes and aptitudes that are different from those of the parents. It is of paramount importance that the parents demonstrate that they recognise this, and that they validate for the child how he is different from them in these respects – thus aiding the process of the child becoming able to see himself as a person in his own right.

The ongoing understanding of a child's perceptions is in itself a complex subject. At each successive stage in his development, there is an increase in a child's ability to perceive what is around him in the same way as is generally agreed in the society into which he was born. A parent's ability to be able to see and understand things *through the eyes of their child* is fundamental to the ability to help the child to feel truly known by the parent and to make sense of what surrounds him. It is only through this process that a child can progress to the next stage of interfacing confidently with the world around him.

If sufficient understanding of his perceptions is not demonstrated, then the child only has the option of *appearing* to progress, while in truth, he is *performing a role* rather than becoming himself.

Eventually, the new person will become aware of being able to perceive elements of his parents' personalities and psyche *that the parents cannot yet see for themselves*. Parents can find such perceptions quite challenging at times, and may respond with denial rather than demonstrating an ability or a willingness to reflect upon what is being put in front of them. Roald Dahl's book *The Witches* gives us some insight into the child's dilemma when feeling that there is something else behind the apparently plausible mask that is being presented to him. As the child grows and matures, to him at times a parent might actually look different – almost a different person. Examples of this might happen quite suddenly, and the child might feel temporarily disturbed, requiring the reassuring presence of the parent while he discovers that the parent is actually the person he always knew him or her to be. Experiencing the changing roles, and 'faces', of a parent are an inevitable part of the process of maturation of a new person through childhood.

As part of the long slow process of separation, the child will gradually become aware that his parents cannot provide everything. This is an essential stage in the process of separation. The parents must aspire to provide *sufficiently* in both the physical and the emotional arenas, but they cannot provide *everything*. If *sufficient* is being provided and is received by the child, the child is then in a position where he can choose to take in *additional* input from other appropriate adult sources. Part of adequate parenting involves encouraging children to rely upon a range of trustworthy people by whom they and their parents are known. In the process of recruiting such people – *significant others* – into a child's life, it is of prime importance that the child can observe *positive links* between such people and his parents, within which information about the child is shared and transmitted.

Early elements of the separation process include the child being helped to reach the stage where he can see mother go out *to be somewhere where he is not*. Another is the child knowing and understanding that mother has people she interacts with who are *not him*. A child's capacity to reach the point where he does not experience such situations as being disturbing, or as a threat, depends upon the central parent's ability to demonstrate that he or she is there for him – whether or not physically present or in direct interaction. The creation and ongoing evolution of a *close confiding relationship* between child and parent is fundamental to this.

In the early years, it is quite common for mother and child to employ the use of particular cuddly toys, special ribbons or blankets. The favoured item becomes instilled with the same meaning as the sense of close connection with the parent. Such items are sometimes known as *transitional objects*. By carrying the 'message of close connection' their existence forms a bridge between the physical presence and physical absence of the parent.

Games that involve the parent disappearing for but a moment, only to re-emerge, with a smile and a cuddle, provide more of the many helpful approaches that aid the process of the small child becoming able to grasp that the parent still exists even when out of sight. The parent's voice calling the child's name from a nearby room or singing a familiar song are further examples of this. A more evolved version is for a trusted parent substitute, who is caring for the child for an hour or so, to take the child to a previously-agreed meeting place to 'find Mummy'.

Having reached the point where he is sure enough that the mother person is there for him, the child slowly discovers more and more about the world, including who the mother person is *as well as* being the satisfier of his needs.

'Separation'

What if the parents of a child decide to live separately?

The first thing to remember is that you chose your partner, and you chose to live with that person and create a child together. The child is not in the same position. The child is the embodiment of a creative act between two people. In essence the child does not have a choice to rid himself of one or the other of those people.

When living with one parent who is unhappy about the presence of the other, the child may well seem to agree with one or the other parent. The child may even appear to fit in with the 'lure' of the thought of having two bedrooms – one in each of the parents' new homes. But what the child really wants and needs is for his parents to be in the same dwelling, behaving as a united parent couple. He needs to have ease of access to both these people, as a child needs the interaction with each of them and both of them together as the baseline in relation to which he grows and develops as a human being.

The ongoing interaction of a boy with his father gives him a baseline template from and through which he will view other males in society. And he also needs the ongoing interaction with his father so that he can discover himself as a male person in his own right. In the early years, a male child will identify with his father, and copy him. But as he grows and matures, the father and son notice not only the similarities between them, but also the ways in which they are dissimilar. This is the basis from which the son begins to discover his separate identity. It is important that the father is as interested in the differences as he is in the similarities between them. This interest helps to validate the development of his son's separate identity. Shared interest in life around them forms an essential part of their developing friendship, which can lead to a lifelong adult friendship.

A boy's identification with his mother is different. She is the first example of a female that he will know, and her position around him and interaction with him provide a template from and through which he will view other females in society.

A child's relationship with his parents as a couple allows that child to interact with his origins, and also provides a template from and through which the child views relationships between other parent couples. Together and as individuals, the parents provide and develop a springboard from which the child can reach out into life.

A daughter's main identification is with her mother. For a boy or a girl to manifest as merely a carbon copy of the personality of the mother, the father, or a combination of both, is not a good outcome, as the unique personality of that new person would have been obscured, or worse, snuffed out.

A young person who has been helped to discover his own personality is someone who can connect securely and confidently with other people. He is a person who can search for and discover his path through adult life, manifesting as someone who is distinct from his origins.

Some other important aspects of separation

A well known psychoanalyst, Lily Pincus, wrote of a couple who when they came to see her said, 'Help us to separate so that we can live together.' These people had realised that there was something happening in their relationship which meant that too many of their interactions were not based on two people discussing things with one another – thus creating endless unhelpful and confusing 'tangles'. They knew that if they could see and understand what was happening to them, continuing living together would become possible. It was necessary to look at unresolved problems from their early lives – thus enabling them to see what they were really trying to express, and to whom.

It is almost universal that at times each of us finds ourselves addressing our spouse or partner in a way that stems entirely from something that was missing or wrong in the early years of our life. If not enough of the true separation process has taken place in relation to the parents or their representatives, then the offspring person is at risk of finding themselves struggling in the interactive processes with a partner in adult life – in ways that are confusing to both of them, and are of no help to either of them. This is because the sufferer is not really speaking to the partner, but to someone who is not there. The presence of the partner is used for this purpose. Even when the basis of the problem can be identified as having originated from a particular time or pattern from childhood years, the sufferer still has to develop an objective and clear grasp of it. Only then can he explain to a bemused partner where distortions in his approach have come from. If both members of the couple have such problems, then the resulting confusion can take quite some time to disentangle!

In recent years, it has become increasingly apparent that people who were created from donor semen, anonymously provided, are vulnerable to feelings of incompleteness and emptiness, and a sense that something is missing. This has led to a change in the law, so that anonymous donation is no longer accepted in the UK. In order to develop and mature into a full adult person, a child does need more than being given a physical body and being nurtured solely by a mother person.

The provisions of the Family Law (Scotland) Act 2006 cover the need of the child to see his father. Any child born after the date of the commencement of the Act has a legal right to see his father, and is enabled in this.

How can things be managed when a parent is ill? If the parent remains at home, then the child can be helped to interface with the new situation, which everyone would hope is temporary. If the illness cannot be managed at home, then the child has to face the physical absence of that parent. Not only is the parent not there, but also feelings of anxiety and distress are attached to that absence. Talking to the child about the absent parent is essential, whatever illness is involved, and however worried the adults might be.

The child's ability to keep the ongoing knowledge of his parent alive in his inner structure can be seriously impaired or disrupted by this kind of enforced separation, unless there is sufficient conversation about that parent going on around him, and with him. If there is a total disruption in the sense of connection that the child has with the parent, then how that parent relates to the child later about his or her absence is crucial. The parent must be able to demonstrate that he grasps how the child must have been feeling in his absence, and he must be prepared to repeat that understanding as often as is necessary to validate the child's reality, thus enabling the child to reconnect securely with him.

Separation by death is a permanent loss. It is a situation where a child has to rely upon those who know both him and the deceased person for the development of his understanding of why that person is no longer there and how he feels about that loss.

While attending lectures on forensic medicine, I met a fiscal depute who at that time was dealing with case material involving deaths. I learned that one of her parents was Russian, and that this meant she had lived in Russia during her early years. She had clear memory of the 'open casket' system there, where she, and any other friend or relative of the deceased, could view the body in a coffin in the home environment. For her, this, combined with the attitudes of those around her in those years, had left her with no fears or discomfort about a dead body. This is one important aspect of loss through death. The other one of central importance is the feeling that the relationship has been severed. This severance can be bridged, but only if those who knew that person continue to talk about him, in a way that demonstrates that he lives on in their minds, and that they have an understanding of the child's grief. A child needs the adults around him to be like this, so that he, too, can remain consciously connected with the knowledge of the deceased person.

How can a person parent a child through such loss when also being severely impacted upon by that loss? This requires an honesty and openness, appropriate to the age and stage of development of the child, to evolve hand in hand with the parent's or carer's own grieving process.

77

A very interesting example of an unusual issue of separation was televised some years ago, when female Siamese twins, around one year old, were about to be separated surgically. They were joined at the chest, and shared some of their internal structures. I remember seeing the mother playing with her joined daughters, using a Siamese twin doll which was constructed in a way that it could be pulled apart into two dolls.

Very sadly, only one of the twins survived, so that twin not only lost part of her own body, but also her conjoined sister. She never had the chance to get to know her sister from a separate body, and she needed help to lay down the seeds of a grieving process for that loss.

'Separation anxiety'

I have used quote marks around the term above, as I often do not feel comfortable about its usage in many contexts. At worst, it might be applied as a kind of criticism – either of a child or of his parent. Nearly as bad is its use as a kind of 'diagnosis' – i.e. 'he is suffering from separation anxiety', stated as if this were an illness.

If we consider some reasons why a child might feel anxious when he is about to be parted from his parent or when he is away from the parent, and look into what might be done to help this kind of situation, the outcome is likely to be helpful all round.

During the long slow process of a child evolving into a separate human being with his own unique identity, there are many times when the child has to be somewhere where the parent is not. Physical safety in such situations can be ensured by protected environments and staff who are trained adequately, or the presence of trusted friends or relatives. Emotional disturbance can present in the form of 'clinging' 'anxious' behaviour on the part of the child if there are not sufficient prompts present in his environment that link him to the ongoing knowledge of the existence of the parent.

Such prompts habitually include a familiar setting with familiar people, but there may be certain particular items that for a child carry intense meaning of ongoing connection with the parent. These 'transitional objects' are often a teddy bear, other favourite stuffed toy or a special blanket. The variations on this theme are endless, and can include promises of what will take place when parent and child are reunited – hugs, reading a story from a special book and so on.

There may be very specific things that a child needs to communicate to a parent before being apart. Many such matters can be easily guessed at, but others may take time to unravel. If the parting is imminent, and unravelling time is not then available, a cast-iron promise of when a special chat can take place can be made to tide the child over the separation.

I once knew a girl who, at four years of age, was excited about starting nursery. However, each time her mother took her to the school nursery, the girl clung to her desperately and would not let her go. Despite the advice of the staff to leave her there, the mother would calmly take her home again.

The mother was correct in what she did. She had adopted this child a year earlier, and from her knowledge of her background, she knew that she had been 'handed over' several times. To this girl, 'being handed over' meant 'never getting back home again'. She needed a situation where the mother person would accept her panic, and be with her in it. Only then would the girl be able to move into the position where she could believe that her home and her mother person would be there again for her after being apart.

Situations do exist where it is the parent's anxiety that holds a child back, and these require sensitive investigation. 'Labelling' of the parent does not help to elucidate what the problem actually is.

I heard the following example of a pattern of anxiety many years ago, and it has remained etched in my mind ever since.

A friend's sister had adopted two sons who, at that time, were attending primary school. One of the boys suffered from chronic severe asthma, and his adoptive mother was watchful and concerned about this.

One day, the boys were to be left with my friend while their mother went to deal with a lengthy errand. As soon as she left, the asthmatic boy started to wheeze intensely.

My friend, impatient with some aspects of her sister's attitude to this boy's asthma, turned to him and said, 'Stop that at once! Auntie doesn't like it!'

Immediately, the boy stopped wheezing, and there was no return of this affliction during his stay with his aunt. He behaved in a relaxed, happy way.

It seemed to me that there was some kind of 'feedback loop' taking place between the asthmatic child and the adoptive mother, where each was taking part in perpetuating the loop. It was not a situation where I felt I could ask anything about the surrounding circumstances. However, I imagine that the adoptive mother might well have carried considerable anxiety about the health of the children who had come into her care, and that this may have been one of the triggers to the bouts of wheezing that the asthmatic boy experienced. When his aunt made it clear that he did not need to wheeze for her, he was temporarily relieved of a certain burden, and laid it to one side.

I am not saying here that all asthmatic attacks stem from a similar kind of cause.

'Sore tummy'

I expect that most parents will be familiar with the cry of 'sore tummy!' This may indeed signal that the child is experiencing pain in the general area of his stomach, but 'sore tummy' is also commonly used as a generic term for any abdominal pain. In fact, such terminology can persist throughout adult life – where a sufferer is unable to distinguish between stomach pain and other abdominal pains, such as from the transverse colon.

Any expression of pain must, of course, be taken seriously, as it is important to identify what is actually happening. Physical pain may require prompt input from a medical professional. However, the term 'sore tummy' can be a cry for help about something else.

A child will soon learn that 'sore tummy' is language for a much broader spectrum of distress. If he is feeling uncomfortable, and his parent notices this, the question 'Have you got a sore tummy?' might be one of the first to be asked. In fact, even before a child is able to speak, he will hear his parent remark to others 'Perhaps he's got a sore tummy' when pondering upon the child's unsettledness. In this kind of way a 'sore tummy currency' can be established quite early in life.

Consequently, it is relatively easy for a child to equate a painful emotional state with 'sore tummy'. After all, emotional pain is often experienced as if it were hurting inner organs such as the heart and the intestines. This is not surprising, as the autonomic nervous system that provides the nerve supply to such organs and organ systems is easily affected by emotional disturbance.

Later, specific anxiety about going somewhere where the parent is not (e.g. school) can manifest as 'sore tummy'. This can be for several reasons, which are very likely to be interconnected.

The child might be anxious about being away from the parent if there is something important to him that he has not yet been able to communicate to the parent. The reader will see an example of this portrayed in 'A Story of Tim' that appears at the end of this book. Tim's anxiety about not knowing where his parents will be is troubling him. This is addressed appropriately.

Brushing such anxiety to one side can lead to a weakening of a child's essential attachment to his parents, whereas treating it so seriously that the parents do not go out after all can risk adding to the child's feelings of anxiety. Finding a way of perpetuating a sense of connection between the parents and the child while the parents are out enables the child to embrace a new situation. Tim could have complained about a 'sore tummy' if his mother had not interacted with him appropriately. Apart from using 'sore tummy currency' he may well have had painful gripping sensations in his abdomen. However, those feelings are likely to have faded had she then focused on the emotional disturbance rather than the cries about physical pain.

Any parent would be well advised to take all possible elements into account when presented with a 'sore tummy' child.

'Sore ears' are a different matter. A pre-verbal or newly verbal child who seems restless, unhappy, perhaps a little hot, and who might tug at one or the other ear is a child who needs a medical professional to check his ears for any infection.

When my children were small, I rapidly came to the conclusion that if in doubt about the presence or absence of an ear infection, the best thing was to get the ears checked. I decided that even if on occasion I appeared foolish to the medical profession, the risks inherent in not discovering the presence of an ear infection were too high. I was glad to encounter one particular GP, who had four daughters and felt exactly the same way as I did.

Significant others

To the baby, Mother is everything, but this situation does not last forever. If the mother's life is such that she can remain sufficiently consistently and freely available to her baby, he uses this at-one-ness as the central anchor to his reality, and he will slowly begin to be able to assimilate other experiences as being meaningful to his life.

In modern times, it is not uncommon for the main person in a baby's life to be someone other than the birth mother. For example, the father might take up the 'mother' position. Similarly, a grandparent or an aunt may do so.

The 'mother' must be someone who has the same attachment potential to the new human being as the birth mother would have. That is, it must be someone whose inner structure is linked strongly and reliably to the physical and emotional wellbeing of the infant – enabling him to have that feeling of at-one-ness with the 'mother person' that he would have with his actual mother.

The foundation of an infant's life outside the womb is laid in such a relationship. The central relationship is one of primary attachment. If this relationship is secure and reliable enough, then the infant can begin to embrace other relationship experiences, adding the meaning of them to the baseline of his life, which is his attachment to a mother person.

If the primary relationship is not present consistently enough, the infant has to endure a state of agitation. In the early months, his world disappears when his relationship with the anchor person is disrupted, and his experience is that he ceases to exist. His normal response to this is to scream and scream and scream.

If the disruption continues for long enough, then slowly the infant moves into mute despair. Many years ago, when the parents of infants and small children in hospital were discouraged from visiting, this state of mute despair was misinterpreted as the child having 'settled'. In the 1960s James and Joyce Robertson filmed exactly how that 'settling' came about, with all its initial stages of emotional torment clearly demonstrated. (See 'Other reading'.)

If a central attachment is not laid down and maintained, the consequences are many and varied. I will give two examples – one from each end of the spectrum of possibilities. A child who has lost all hope of attachment can become entirely inturned, at worst unable to recognise human relationship at all. He may be found sitting in a corner, engaged in endlessly repetitive actions such as twisting a finger through his hair. At the other end of the spectrum, a child who, despite the absence of a central attachment, is still affected by the inner driving force of the need to be involved with a person for fundamental attachment to life and relationships, can run excitedly to *any* person, greeting any stranger as if he or she were the central person.

Twins each require a unique and individual relationship with the mother person. If this is not developed, then there can be a high risk that the main attachment of each twin is to the other, and not to the mother person. In the most extreme cases, the twins then live a life that is turned inwards, including only the other as being relevant, and excluding other people and the rest of life. Identical twins are more vulnerable in this respect.

A loving grandmother might provide consistent care for an infant, relating to her grandchild as devotedly as if he were her own. This can be a truly wonderful situation, but we should remember that the child's experience and reality must be relayed back to the mother, and in a way that the child can absorb. If not, the child runs the risk of perceiving the grandmother in his emotional structure as if she were the actual mother. If this is the case, then the eventual loss of the grandmother through death is complex. To the child, experientially he has lost his mother, whereas to his family and to society at large, he has lost a grandparent. Unless this is understood and accepted, the grief process cannot proceed in the way that it needs to. This concept remains true even if by the time of the loss, the child has become an adult.

I was once speaking to a Nigerian man who was in his thirties. He told me something of the culture in which he had been brought up. I found it fascinating to learn that although he knew who his birth parents were, he was taught to call all adults of that age group 'Mummy' or 'Daddy' and that all these people had responsibility as parent people to all the youngsters. He described how everyone in the extended family ate from the same communal bowls, and visitors who were passing through knew that they could roll out a mat in any communal home.

The demeanour of this man struck me as being calm and quietly confident. Everything he said and did came from basic human common sense and collaborative ethos. He carried himself with natural dignity.

Another example of the benefits of communal living became apparent to me when I visited a friend who lived in a religious community where most of the adults were involved in ordinary everyday jobs. The children in this community emanated a sense of confidence, and ran from building to building, never in any doubt about the reception that they would receive. They radiated a natural maturity in the way that they interacted with adults and with one another.

I remember seeing a book of old photographs of scenes from Falkirk of many years ago. One of these has stayed in my mind, never very far away from my consciousness. It is of a row of stone-built terraced flats, with an external access stairway at each end. On the steps of one of these stairways had gathered all the occupants of the flats, and the ease between them was clearly apparent. They could all have been from one happy family, although I was certain that genetically they were not.

In such communal settings, the children are surrounded by 'significant others', all of whom know their birth parents and everyone else very well.

I am not in any way saying that all communal settings are ideal for the raising of children. Some have their own potential for laying down layers of damage in their young. However, the ones I have mentioned clearly did not, and the children benefited greatly from the plentiful and probably inexhaustible supply of 'significant others'.

'Significant others' are people who are important to the new person in his early years *in addition to the mother person*. These people might be relatives, friends or neighbours. Each has an important role to play in that each brings something to the child that can enrich his life by *adding to what he is already receiving*. It is important that the child can see a positive connection between such people and his mother person. If there is dissonance in the relationship between the mother person and the other person, this can set up conflict inside the small person.

Significant others such as nannies, *au pair* helpers, childminders, and later, teachers, are not usually from the same genetic origins as their charges. However, such people often take the place of the birth parents, temporarily and to varying degrees. In these roles it is essential that a viable link between them and the birth parents is demonstrated in daily life, so that the children hear them talking with the birth parents about the events of the day and how the children felt, and know that they can join in with any such discussion. The children need to see that these other people who are so closely involved in their care are at ease in their relationship with the birth parents. Although a less intense need than the one for being able to observe collaboration between the birth parents, it is nonetheless extremely important. The child's need for this is the same in relation to step-parents and other 'acquired relatives'.

Many years ago, when my children were small, we had a friend whose two children were a little younger. The older of them, a boy, was pleased when he could come to play at our house, away from his little sister.

When his mother came to collect him, he would shout at her from the door, 'Go away! I want Uzzer Mummy!' Uzzer Mummy was, of course, me. Well, it was nice to know that he liked me, but far more important was that his connection with his own mother was supported and sustained. I would tell him that it had been nice to see him here, and that he could come and play with us again, but that now it was time to go home with Mummy. He would scream angrily. Of course, he *was* angry, and there was no way round that. He had to have his angry feelings, and it was important for us to be accepting of that. His calm relaxed state in my home with me and my children had been disrupted by the arrival of his mother and his baby sister, and he was very angry indeed about that. The birth of his baby sister had been a big challenge to him, and, returning to his home environment, he was still consumed by his need to express his rage about it.

'Difficult' relatives may engage with a child in a way that deliberately provokes disturbance in the relationship between the child and his mother person. This is potentially damaging, as it can create inner conflict for the child, and can isolate him from his trusting relationship with his central anchor.

There are some people who, driven by their own unmet infant needs, can be unhelpful towards the parent of a young child, or, worse, can be actively undermining to the parent. Such dynamics can appear in the relationship between grandparents and the parents of the child. They can also manifest from other relatives, or from 'well-meaning friends'. Such approaches can be severely undermining towards the parents' loving relationship with their child. They can also be undermining of the parents' confidence in their parenting role.

On observing a loving attentive mother relating to her child, the hidden deprived child inside the adult relative or friend can counsel: 'You're making a rod for your back by giving him so much attention.' Or such a relative or friend might vie for the parent's attention by talking incessantly, or constantly steering any dialogue away from the needs of the young child. In contrast, a sufferer of early deprivation who has some objective grasp of his situation might say, 'When I see you nursing your baby, I can feel sad and empty because of what I didn't have myself.' And the mother might reply, 'I'm so sorry you didn't get what you needed when you were small. Tiny people are so vulnerable and need a lot of help.' In this way, the sufferer's pain is expressed, and he receives a compassionate response. The interaction is real and truthful, and allows a feeling of closeness and meaning to grow from it.

Note:

Children may not necessarily perceive grandparents and other significant people in the same way as the parents do. This can be so *even if they speak as if that is the case.* It is important to enable sharing of views and perceptions about other people, and to allow the possibility of reviewing these along the way.

Food

At a large supermarket, I saw a cylindrical form of processed meat in the cold meat counter. It had a smiling face on its cutting surface, created by a variation in the colour of the meat product. A small child in a trolley saw it. He pointed to it and looked at his mother. The mother shared with him an interest in it.

Such meat products contain preservative in the form of nitrites. I understand that the average deterioration time of a modern dead human body is slower than in the past, before such preservatives were added to food.

How can a parent protect a child from this kind of situation? A child likes to see the smiling face. The smiling face is in a display of food. The mother is someone who endorses and validates the presence of smiling faces in other contexts – such as happiness amongst people and drawings of smiles. Can a young child distinguish between a smile in the right place and a smile in the wrong place?

I think that the best I could have done in that situation would have been to say, 'Oh, yes, I can see a smiley face', before going on to complete my shopping away from the display.

In an era when there is a lot of worry about people whose bodies have become weighed down by extra stores of fat, many of us try our best to ensure that we and our children eat sensibly.

The plethora of all-day eating places that surround us is a constant reminder to eat. There are places which provide wholesome food, but there are many that do not. How do we guide our children through this maze?

So many people in our culture reach for what they have been

led to believe that they should want, and not what they actually need. How can we relate to our children in a way that results in their not being affected by the subliminal grooming created by the advertising industry?

I noticed in a recent newspaper article that the advice of a senior advisor on food and diet had included the need to allow ourselves 'treats'. But what are treats?

Many years ago, a child might be given a small bar of chocolate on a rare family outing, or perhaps be given a piece of one that was being shared out at a weekend. Such a commodity would be viewed as a 'treat' – something that was different from the everyday. I am concerned about how the concept of a 'treat' has moved into an arena where something that was never an everyday item can now be consumed almost daily, and in large quantities.

It is crucial that we enable our children to distinguish between wholesome food and matter that has been 'dressed up' to provoke consumption. The former is for nourishment and the latter is for the income of the manufacturer and the likelihood of extra expense to us all in the form of increased burden on the NHS.

Some years ago, I watched a programme that a friend had asked me to view. I remember seeing three girls around the age of ten being interviewed. Two of them were smartly dressed and were slender. The third wore comfortable, unremarkable clothes, and carried some extra weight. When interviewed, the 'thin' girls said that they thought about weight and body shape every day, and that it concerned them. When asked about her thoughts, the other girl considered for a moment before replying that her mind was normally full of her interests, so that thoughts about body shape were something that ordinarily did not occur to her. I rejoiced at this. Clearly, she came from a situation where family members were interested in her as a whole person, and did not focus undue attention upon her body. She carried herself in a calm, relaxed and naturally self-assured way. The other girls spoke of anxiety. They were concerned about how they 'ought' to appear.

'Comfort eating'

It is not at all uncommon for the above term to be applied to someone who is frequently eating more than is actually required. Sometimes it is the person themselves who uses the term, and sometimes it is a friend or a 'professional'.

In any case, the behaviour to which the term is applied is not really anything to do with comfort. In fact, fundamentally it is a lack of it. The whole situation is one of *dis*comfort. It is because of adverse stressors, such as difficult emotions, that a person reaches for extra food – in a desperate attempt to numb emotional disturbance or pain. And the result of eating a quantity of extra food in itself can often be physically uncomfortable. Consequently, 'discomfort eating' would be a more appropriate term to apply.

In this kind of situation, it is clear that the eater follows the impulse to eat because he *believes* that he will feel better for doing so. And it is that impulse which needs to be examined. It may be the case that at the point of acting upon the impulse and ingesting the food, there is a feeling of well-being, but that feeling is only temporary. In order to perpetuate the feeling, the sufferer needs to ingest more food, and then more, and more. As this continues, the feeling of well-being becomes less and less accessible, and is eventually replaced by one of discomfort.

When a baby is first born it is more or less still an extension of the mother, albeit on the outside rather than the inside of her.

The continuous provision of nourishment in the womb is replaced by some kind of feeding pattern. At one end of the spectrum this might at first be well-nigh continuous breastfeeding, whereas at the other end of the spectrum it could be three-hourly feeds from bottles of milk substitute. In any case, as time goes on, feeds that are provided at intervals appropriate to the baby's requirements gradually form some kind of pattern.

If this is the formative experience of life outside the womb, then it should hardly be surprising that if people feel insecure or upset, quite a number of them will turn instinctively to a feeding experience, expecting that this will calm them. A further consideration in this picture is that breast milk, and therefore also its substitute, is quite sweet. Those who turn to food in a failed attempt to calm themselves often reach for items that are intensely sweet.

Although I accept that there are metabolic reasons why a person might become 'hooked up' on eating sweet things, it is important to understand that the psychological 'drivers' can be very intense indeed. After all, early feeding is not only associated with intense sweetness, but is also connected with the instinct to survive, and this in turn is inextricably connected to the basis of emotional attachment. Hence we are looking at dynamics that are extremely powerful indeed.

While some seek the early memory of emotional security by engaging in a feeding experience, commonly sweet-tasting, others reach for a bottle. Of course the problems can be compounded if that bottle is full of alcohol. And alcohol carries with it its own intrinsic ability to numb all emotions, albeit temporarily.

The long-term effects of eating very sweet commodities on a frequent basis are well documented. The sufferer's bodyweight usually increases, and this alone can lead to stress on tissues and organs. In addition, carbohydrate metabolism can reach the stage where it cannot keep up with what it is being required to do, and the sufferer may begin to exhibit a diabetic state of some degree.

It is not all that long ago in history that sweet things were either not available, or were only available in small quantities and at certain times of the year. Honey has been available for a very long time, but not everyone had access to it, and if they did, it would only be seasonal. Consequently, the ingestion of this relatively rare sweet food was self-limiting.

In modern Western culture, less and less do we have events that lead to limiting of the availability of sweet-tasting things. In fact the reverse has been true, and for many people, more and more is readily accessible, at any time of the day or night. Larger and larger containers of sweets and chocolates have been promoted for sale. Clearly the manufacturers do not have the best interests of their customers at heart! And people can behave as if these enhanced quantities are entirely desirable.

Where sweets are concerned, the use of the concept of a 'treat' can be a snare and a delusion. In our current culture, is it sensible to implant in a child's mind the idea that the eating of sweets is a 'treat' – i.e. something special that is in some way prized?

I am not saying here that children should be protected from consuming sweets. I am only asking that we consider detaching the 'treat' concept from such commodities, as it puts an extra level of emotional significance on them. 'Maybe we could share a bag of sweets at the weekend' does not have the same emotional impact as 'We'll have a wonderful treat tonight!' 'Would you like to choose a sweet out of the bag that Granny left for us?' is quite different from a child being given carte blanche to eat his way through a container of sweets.

Another word that may be applied to the consumption of sweets is 'reward'. The concept of a 'reward' can readily become distorted by such an association.

I do understand that we have to find a way of helping our

children to interface with what they see around them, but supporting them by constructing approaches that aid the development of personal balance is far more helpful than providing extra sweets as 'treats' or 'rewards'.

I have known many people who, while searching for inner calm, look for it in places where it simply cannot be found. The first step in the long process of examining this is to become aware that one might well be 'looking in the wrong cupboards'. Addictive patterns inevitably involve reaching out repetitively for something – the wrong thing – that can never satisfy a craving.

And where can true comfort be found? True comfort arises from the knowledge of relationship that is based on trust. A child who is given a trusting connection with a parent or parent representative is one who, when distressed, reaches out to human relationship for comfort. And that comfort is derived from his manifest distress being recognised and understood, giving it validity and thus confirming the reality of his suffering. Once that begins to happen, the child feels connected to the other person in his distress. The emotion then becomes bearable, and its intensity fades. In later life, such a person is unlikely to reach for false sources of 'comfort'. Instead he connects with other human beings in relationships in which sharing and close confiding are integral parts.

Religion

We live in an era where a considerable number of churches have ceased to be used for worship. At best, such buildings have been transformed into offices, houses or flats. At worst, they lie derelict, and are crumbling. Many places of worship were built on sites that had already been used for worship, either in a previous building or as a recognised gathering place. It is my understanding that people from long ago had a sense of the right place to build – a geographical location and line of construction that had deep meaning and significance in the belief system of the time – and that this would enable worshippers to connect with a greater power, something that was integral with life, and was also beyond it.

The idea of a god-entity has persisted from far back in the development of the human race, and currently manifests in many forms, each of which is entirely meaningful and valid to the daily life of particular groups of people. However, I can see other prominent systems which, although they purport to bring meaning and satisfaction to life, could well be misleading.

I remember the first time that I saw the Trafford Centre, initially from a distance, when driving to Manchester. That glimpse impacted on me in a way that signalled the presence of an extensive and impressive place of worship. Having later decided to visit it, I struggled with the plethora of 'retail units' and the cacophony of noise that emanated from them. To me, the outer appearance of the building belied what it harboured, and I found this quite disturbing. Judging by the number of people visiting it, this was an important gathering place, but my observations of what these people were doing there left me with an overall sense of sadness.

What should we teach our children about religion? If we belong to a particular faith, it is likely that we will encourage our offspring to follow that same path. But what should we do if our own beliefs are unformed or uncertain? Overall, my view would be to introduce our children to the existence of religion and its many forms, as one would aspire to do about any other subject of note. At the very least, an interest in religion is relevant to the understanding of history and a grasp of certain elements of the social structure in which we live.

My personal concern is that if we do not keep the knowledge of religion in balance with the knowledge and experience of other elements of daily life, then the evolution of a child's need to discover his spirituality may be delayed or become stunted. What each of us think spirituality actually is will vary widely, but to keep open a sense of there being something beyond the mundane tasks of daily life, something shared, although named and perceived in many different ways, will help to keep the child's mind open.

Unless children are encouraged to learn about how food is produced and where it comes from, there is a risk that they will think that food originates in a supermarket, frequently in boxes. Without food, none of us could live. Perhaps we could consider transmitting to our children the importance of being thankful that we have access to it? Some would express this by thanking a god-entity for the food. Others might speak out a thought of thanks to the farmers who work so hard, in conditions that can be harsh.

The general atmosphere of the current drive to consume – both food and other commodities – appears to be out of balance with the need to reflect about life and one's part in it. A child's developmental need to identify with his parents or parent figures, and, as he grows, with his peer group, can leave him very vulnerable to absorbing a cultural 'norm' of life revolving around acquiring new things.

We should be particularly concerned that the kind of advertising to which our children are exposed so often relies upon contriving to make people, and children in particular, believe that they cannot feel all right unless they acquire whatever is being promoted. Any lack of a sense of inner security leaves a person vulnerable to imagining 'if only I could have a ... then I would feel all right'. This, coupled with the developmental imperatives of peer group identification, can leave a child or young person wide open to exploitation. Life is not really tenable when conducted as a series of 'quick fixes' and 'getting things'.

Could it be that a trip to a drive-through eating establishment and a visit to the local shopping mall have in part taken the place of worship in a religious belief-system?

The so-called 'celebrity culture' is greatly puzzling. It seems that there is an intense interest in certain people who have considerable sums of money and a particular kind of status, and that the media are heavily involved in this. Could it be that the media have created the intensity of this interest by relying on it as a main focus of reporting?

Mankind has always demonstrated a propensity to find a leader. I imagine that in the past such leaders were people who were big and strong, particularly wise, had some special healing powers, or were religious leaders. Within that frame, can modern 'celebrities' really be experienced as valid 'leaders'?

I had a very interesting discussion with a group of children aged about eleven years, during which one of them asked me if I was a celebrity, and if I had been on television. The purpose of our meeting had been to talk about creative writing, but I felt that it was important to answer these questions. I told them that I did not have celebrity status, but that I had been on television.

Feeling that I wanted to take this line of inquiry further, I then began to ask each of them what jobs their parents did. One boy started to snigger, saying that his mother cleaned toilets. I looked him straight in the eye and said: 'Well, I regard her as being a celebrity. Where would we all be if someone was not prepared to clean the toilets?' I then went on to elucidate the likely outcomes. The result was electrifying. Each child tried to think of a relative who had a job such as street waste collection, the cooking of school meals, and cleaning in offices and hospitals. I continued to validate in detail the fundamental importance of such work.

And what is Christmas? I have found myself wishing many times that there could be an event, known by a different name, in the middle of winter, that is separate from the religious significance of Christmas. The muddle that arises from the lack of separation appears in many contexts, and I cannot think that it is of help or value to our children.

The emotional security that we help our children to build inside themselves should lead to a sense of their being a person in their own right, from which position they can link to others and collaborate with them. Lack of emotional security leaves a child vulnerable to losing his sense of himself to identification with a group or culture, blindly caught up in following the 'norms' and 'requirements' of that particular group, whether or not those norms and requirements foster social cohesion.

It would be very sad indeed to think that our young were being drawn into repetitive ephemeral activities that have little or no sustaining meaning, rather than having their minds open to considerations of the eternal.

Untruth, and the use of partial truth

A parent might lie to his child quite deliberately, or a parent might decide to be conservative with the truth.

In the former case, it is clear that the parent is more concerned about his own comfort than that of the child. Worse, because the parent is the 'safe, trusted' anchor point for the child, the child's central self is being fed on untruth. This is quite different from the situation of an adult person, who, on being told a lie, has other experience from which to assess the veracity of what he is hearing. He has the inner equipment with which to develop an objective overview of what he is being told. The child does not.

In the latter case, the parent may, correctly, be attempting to give the child information that he is sure the child can understand and cope with. However, as the competent parent will realise, such conservatism should be open to regular review – such review taking place over time, as the child grows and matures. It should also take place in response to any further questioning from the child around the time of the initial event.

I think that it is almost invariably the case that subjects which the parent imagines the child will find impossibly difficult are the ones which the parent will find the hardest to address directly and honestly. It is quite common for a parent to be fearful of the child 'being upset' by certain information. It is important to make a distinction between a situation where upset is *caused* to a child, and one where a child *expresses upset* about a situation which is clearly upsetting. This latter case is a healthy and normal part of emotional life, whereas the former might have strayed into an arena where a child is being given information in a wrong way – e.g. too much, too little, or the wrong kind of attitude being manifested by the person who imparts it.

If a child *presents* upset feeling states on hearing about an upsetting situation, then the parent can validate such feelings and offer comfort. Supposing, for example, that Auntie Rose's baby develops a serious illness, and little Fergus, aged three, doesn't yet know about this.

'Mummy, I want to see Auntie and the baby this afternoon.'

'I'm afraid we won't be able to do that. Maybe on another day…'

If little Fergus is satisfied with this, then there is no need at that stage to say anything about the baby's illness. After all, it is likely that the adults themselves do not yet know enough about it.

However, if Fergus persists:

'But I want to see them *today*.'

Then it is important for the mother to say something like:

'Auntie said that the baby isn't feeling well at the moment.'

'But when I'm not feeling well, I like to see Auntie,' Fergus might well reason.

'I know, but the baby's illness is the sort where it's best to be quiet and sleepy for a while.'

If this is not sufficient, the interaction might progress to the point where the mother says that she will be phoning Auntie later on, that she'll say that Fergus is looking forward to seeing her and the baby again soon, and that he's asking how the baby is.

Such an approach can be applied whether the baby is suffering from a fluey cold or whether it is suffering from something more serious. Fergus's wish to see his auntie and the baby is being respected, and he is being included in any conversation with the baby's mother, his aunt.

If the baby has to go to hospital suffering from something like suspected meningitis, Fergus can be told that Auntie is taking the baby to hospital to see some special doctors who will help her to learn more about how to make the baby feel better, and so on.

The above sample dialogue is a template from which anyone can extemporise appropriately. If at any stage Fergus shows distress about the situation, the parent can validate this by saying something like 'I can perfectly understand why you feel upset/angry etc about not being able to see them today. You like them both a lot, and you must be feeling very disappointed.' A hug or two, or a stroking of the back, arm or head can be an integral part of this.

We must also take into account that if the baby is seriously ill, it is not unlikely that Fergus would pick something up from the voice tones of adults, or from things he overhears them saying. In such situations it may well be advisable for the mother to explain that she is feeling worried about the baby. This could be qualified by saying something about how if someone is ill, she often finds herself thinking about them more, hoping that they will get better soon. A suggestion of drawing a picture to give to the baby when it is better will help to focus Fergus's thoughts in a direction which is helpful to both him and the baby.

Early in this sample dialogue, a parent might have been tempted to withhold information about the baby's illness and merely promote the idea that Auntie and the baby are 'busy today'. Such a route might be followed with the best of intentions, but if Fergus later learned that the real reason why he could not see Auntie and the baby that day had been withheld from him, then this is something that could well weaken his trust in those upon whom he depends for his understanding of the world around him.

The temptation to lie to a child about illness can increase greatly if, for example, the mother's own parent is suffering from an illness which is likely to result in death quite soon. The mother might be afraid to speak about it at all. Her fears might stem from her own fear of 'breaking down' in front of the child, or of anything she says resulting her child apparently feeling as awful as she is. The truth of the matter is that the imminent loss of someone significant in one's life *is* a very upsetting situation, and that the upset involved will linger on for many months after the death itself. The child cannot be 'protected' from this – because the upset lives on, around him, impacting upon him. It is better that he is given information that he asks for, and is offered information such as 'Mummy is feeling very sad today because...' Without this he will be wandering round in an atmosphere that he cannot understand, feeling that he cannot make the kind of connection with his mother that he is used to having, and worse, maybe even feeling that it is *because of him* that he is not getting that connection. And if the child has a meaningful relationship with the person who is about to die, there is the need to prepare him for that loss.

On a less painful front, although quite significant, when one of my friends was going back to work after a number of years of being based at home, her children complained.

'Why do you have to go to work, Mummy? We don't like it. We want you to be here.'

She answered that she was going to work to earn pennies so that they could do nice things together like going on holiday. Away from that situation, I asked her to tell them that she was going to work because she liked doing her work, and that she liked being at home with them, but that she liked work as well. Her children needed to know that work was an interesting and positive experience, which was not an alternative to their mother's life with them, and that they continued to be important to their mother when she was away from them, doing something that she enjoyed for its own sake (as well as for any spin-offs such as family holidays).

I should also point out that children can 'know' things without having been given the information verbally. I have come across many examples of this in my life, and the one that I quote most often is as follows.

A family holiday that included a friend of our oldest child required the travelling to be split into two parts. My husband drove a car with the luggage and our youngest child, while I went by train with the other three children. Gazing out of the window, I relaxed while I watched the pleasant scenery fly by. A thought came into my mind of how the brochure entry for the holiday house had mentioned the possibility that babysitting could be arranged. Then I heard the voice of our seven-year-old son from beside me, saying firmly, 'And you don't need to think about getting a babysitter, either!' I can assure the reader that not only had I not spoken, but also I had not moved my lips in any way. We had not been discussing the matter at all, and the brochure was with the luggage in the car.

Sexual matters

In the early years, a child's natural curiosity will lead him to investigate all kinds of things, and male and female sexual parts are no exception – their own sexual parts, and those of the parents as well. The more a parent can respond to this in an ordinary way, the better.

As a culture we have come a long way towards being natural and open with our young about their questions. This is quite different from the sufferings of generations ago, when boys were ordered, in the absence of any sensible explanation, to 'never touch yourself there'. During my own lifetime, change has been heralded and accomplished. The tendency in families of my childhood for parents not only to conceal their bodies from their children, but also to withhold ordinary basic information about physical functions, has given way to an increasing openness.

However, this whole area of life is one in which it is still quite common for parents to be evasive, and this can manifest in a variety of ways. It is crucial to realise that any reticence or evasion on the part of a parent does not originate from the fact that their small son or daughter is asking questions about relevant body parts, the functioning of these, and any associated emotional states. It is perfectly normal for children to be curious about anything and everything, and sexual matters are no exception.

I would ask any parent to consider the fact that if sexual relating had not taken place, then the child himself would not be there to ask any questions. Why should a child be denied access to information about his very origins?

Any discomfort suffered by the parent arises from their own baseline experience of learning about sexual matters. If parents, as children, were responded to evasively about sexuality, the result can easily be that feelings of discomfort were generated by such a lack of straightforward interaction. Such feelings can then linger on, unchanged, ready to surface when the next generation of children ask the same kind of questions.

It is important that, wherever possible, our children learn about procreation from the two people who created them, and that this information is imparted in a context where real love and respect is manifest. There is no question that parents should encourage children to clean their teeth every day, using a toothbrush and paste of good quality. With adequate care, teeth can even last for a lifetime. Yet there is still hesitance and resistance on the subject of imparting information about sexual matters. How can this be, when the perpetuation of human life depends upon it?

I once asked two senior police officers what their parents had told them about where they had come from. They could not look at me, and appeared to be very uncomfortable. I tried to help them by suggesting that gooseberry bushes or cabbage patches might have been involved, but the whole thing was too much for them.

As with any other subject, a child's questions about sexual matters need to be answered in a way in which he can best incorporate any new material. If in doubt, we should choose a level which is slightly below his conceptual abilities, and he can ask further questions then, or later.

A child might ask some very direct questions indeed. If uncertain about how to respond, the parent may decide to validate the questions and then give some idea of when an answer will be provided. For example, the parent might say 'That's an interesting question...' and add 'we could have a chat about it at bathtime.'

A child who has learned that Mummy and Daddy do something together to make a baby may understandably assume that this action takes place on one occasion for each baby that is born. It depends upon the age of the child, his stage of development and his level of interest in the subject as to whether or not a parent might go on to say that Mummy and Daddy do that thing together at other times, too.

Each child has his own individual way of asking questions, and this will have arisen from the context in which he is growing up. There is no set pattern that dictates when or how questions about sexual parts and sexuality will emerge, particularly in the early years, when the impact of factors external to the family is not so pronounced. Of course, there is the game of Doctors and Nurses, where preschool children will find a place out of sight of the parents and 'examine' one another. In my view it is important to allow such a context and at the same time be sufficiently a part of it. With some thought and reflection, a parent can quickly develop the skill of monitoring the game appropriately.

I remember thinking right from the beginning of the lives of my own children that it could well be wrong for them if I concealed things from them that had been withheld from me. Nakedness and bodily functions were no exception. I remember how this resulted in considerable challenge for me at times. For example, I recall quite vividly the trail of small children and their friends who would follow me to the bathroom and solemnly hand pieces of toilet paper to me to 'help'.

When pregnant with my second child, I extended trips with my firstborn to the antenatal examinations into more comprehensive outings, so that he and I could have a 'day out' during which my examination would take place. I noticed that some nursing staff could be quite uncomfortable about my son being able to see what was being done to me, and would try to 'shield' him from it. I thought this to be strange. After all, the place that they were hiding from him was the place through which he had made his entry to the world. I remember how he was very interested to watch when the stitches were removed from my perineum a few days after the birth of his brother. The nurse who carried this out was completely relaxed about his involvement, and I valued this greatly.

During my pregnancy with the baby who turned out to be a sister for our boys, I employed the use of an old stethoscope so that they could hear their sibling's heartbeat *in utero*. This gave them a broader experience than the observation of my swelling abdomen coupled with the chats about the baby that was growing inside it.

If a child is confident and trusting in his relationship with his parents, he will develop an integrated sense of what close relationship is really about. Using this formative experience of secure relationship as a base, he will know what he feels comfortable with, and will be able to articulate this. He will have the inbuilt ability to differentiate between things that make sense and things that do not. If something does not make sense to him he will question it, and will have the instinct and impulse to refer it back to a trusted parent. This means that the child's actions and reactions are of the kind that keeps him safe. Attempts by potential abusers to coerce such a child into agreeing to engage in an unfamiliar activity are unlikely to succeed.

As I have already stated, if at all possible, it is best that children learn about sexual matters from the people who created them, in a loving environment. That is not to say that 'sex education' in schools is not of value. Teacher-led peer-group discussion can allow a broader perspective to be developed, and for those whose parents find themselves unable to discuss sexuality and sexual functioning, it is invaluable.

Many years ago there was a primary school sexual assault prevention teaching programme for children that was entitled: 'Feeling yes, feeling no'. This programme provided an excellent base from which much could be aired and discussed. Children were encouraged to begin by considering what they liked in ordinary interactions and what they disliked, and how to communicate about this. The accompanying song 'My body's nobody's body but mine, You run your own body let me run mine' is simple and very effective in reminding every child of his actual position.

Medical examinations and procedures, and also visits to a dentist, can often involve exceptions to the rule of a child being encouraged to refuse to do what he does not feel comfortable with. Because of this, it is important to help the child to develop an awareness and understanding of why these situations can be different from interactions in the rest of his life.

I remember very well the first time that my daughter, then about seven years old, had to have a sample of blood taken. The way that the medical staff talked to her to prepare her for the procedure was faultless. I was deeply impressed. Then the sequence moved on to the point where she was asked if they could go ahead and take some blood. She agreed, but the moment that the needle was inserted in her arm, she was clearly horrified. At this point the staff were not so competent. Someone said, in disapproving tones 'But you agreed.' I looked straight at my daughter and said, 'I know you agreed, but you're having a completely normal reaction to having a needle stuck into your arm. Don't worry, it's okay, you're doing fine.' Although I could sense an 'atmosphere' around me, I continued to validate my daughter's reality for her. I knew that that was the most important thing to do at the time. Before we left, we thanked the medical staff for their help. And on the way home, we talked a lot about what had happened.

In adult sexual intimacy, the removal of clothes and the meeting of expanses of bare skin are likely components. In infancy, skin-to-skin contact is a daily reality, but beyond that time, such contact dwindles, and may terminate once it is no longer necessary to be bathed by a parent. Consequently, adult sexual intimacy can provide a sudden and strong reminder of infancy. Because of this, together with feelings of adult sexual arousal, it can prompt to consciousness intense feelings from that time. However, the adult participants in sexual intimacy may not realise that this is the case, and may attribute the feelings that they are experiencing solely to the present-day relationship. Such a lack of awareness is not necessarily problematic. However, if the 'infant-mother' relationship has been problematic, unresolved emotional disturbance from that time can surface into the adult-adult intimacy. Likewise, if sufficient integration to true separateness as a person has not taken place, this can provoke difficulty in the 'present-day' closeness.

And what do you say to your sixteen-year-old daughter who has just told you that she is pregnant? The precise answer to this is not a simple one to construct. However, whatever the struggles of the parent, their initial response should never be angry or aggressive. Whatever the circumstances, the daughter needs the parent to receive the fact that she is carrying a new human life, for which she has responsibility. She needs to know that however difficult things are, the parent will try to stand by her in whatever way is appropriate.

Very sadly, I have known situations where a pregnant teenager has been berated and vilified, thus leaving a lasting scar on her experience of procreation. I have even known of parents who, having behaved thus, later go on to be irresponsible in the area of their own sexual intimacy, and then expect their existing children to be heavily involved in the care of any progeny that comes from their misplaced activities.

'Falling' pregnant...

It used to be that if a woman became pregnant outside marriage, she was deemed to be a 'fallen woman'. The man who was the co-creator of the pregnancy was usually not mentioned. Certainly he was not referred to as a 'fallen man'.

Although pregnancy outside marriage is no longer deemed to create fallen women, I do often hear the words: '[name] fell pregnant' or '[name] has fallen pregnant'. I do not ever get the impression that whoever is speaking is intending to convey the idea that the pregnant woman is a 'fallen woman' in the same frame as in days gone by.

In an era where our society aspires to use 'politically correct' language and terminology that supports 'equality' and aims to remove discrimination, why does this particular use of words persist? And although I have heard several couples refer to the pregnancy of the woman as 'we are pregnant', I have never heard of a man who has 'fallen pregnant'.

To me '[name] is pregnant', '[name] has become pregnant' or '[name] is expecting a baby' are appropriate forms of reference.

'No'

It is fundamental that each child recognises the word 'no', and is helped to understand the meanings of it. There are several.

Most importantly there is a particular use of 'no' that has to carry with it a tone and a demeanour to create a message that halts the child straight away. It is a command. Any child must be helped to recognise this instantly. In effect, it is a communication that means 'STOP!', and must only be used for reasons of immediate safety. A child might need to be halted in his tracks because he is about to stumble into a situation that will cause him physical harm, or because he is behaving in a way that risks inviting physical harm to himself or causing physical harm to another. We should also take into account that a child's interaction with animals can require sudden, unequivocally firm intervention.

In cases such as those outlined above, there is no time to explain anything. The child has to be stopped, and the explanations must take place later. With very young children, such explanations can be provided by 'acting' the dangerous situation as a kind of story or play, so that the child can be helped to see it from the outside. The facts of the story can be told time and time again, and to a range of other people, to enable the child to understand.

A small child whose home is at the entrance to a cul-de-sac, where he can see through the window that older children play there regularly, will assume that he can join them. What he does not realise is that the older children are alert to the dangers of cars and vans. He may try to escape from his house and garden to be with the other children. Supposing one day the garden gate is not properly secured, and he runs out just as a van approaches, signalling to turn into the cul-de-sac. If the parent cannot reach him in time, that parent needs to be certain that if he shouts 'no!' the child will stop.

A small child might have a baseline experience with a dog, perhaps belonging to a relative, that climbing on a dog is great fun. If one day at a play park a strange dog runs up, the child might understandably expect to have the same kind of experience. A parent may well need to be able to stop the child by the use of the word 'no!' from a few yards away, giving him time to reach the child and explain that this dog might not like that kind of playing.

Last summer I was out for a walk. I did not have a coat with me, but I had an umbrella. I had not expected bad weather, but when I was near the next village, which is about two miles away from my home, a heavy shower of rain suddenly began. The protection that my elderly umbrella afforded was inadequate. A group of young girls who must have lived nearby called across to me, instructing me to go home quickly because I was getting very wet. I was impressed by this. It was obvious to me that these girls had been taught to consider issues of safety and wellbeing.

A parent using the word 'no' in a more drawn-out, sustained way, together with turning his head from side to side in the classic 'no' body gesture, is often employed when a child is about to engage, or has just begun to engage, in an action that isn't immediately dangerous, but is not acceptable. Examples of this are 'smearing Mummy's lipstick across the wallpaper' and 'dropping things into the toilet'. Lipstick is like a special crayon that Mummy uses on her face, so why not use it on the lovely big space on the wall? And big people drop things into the toilet every day...

Having deterred a small person from wrecking the new wallpaper, the parent can involve the child in the correct use of the lipstick, or provide something else that produces a bright colour, but on a pad of paper. Regular kindly explanations about how only certain things go down the toilet, and providing games such as 'dropping clothes into the washing basket' should eventually help to modify any potential disabling of the sewage system.

The parent has to be prepared to use physical action to prevent the child from continuing with the unwanted activity. 'No' (meaning 'not this') coupled with a firm, kindly holding of the body or hand of the child, in preparation for redirecting the child's focus, is a useful combination.

The parent who employs a forceful use of the word 'no' but is not ready to follow this up with physical action can find that the effect of his approach may well be quite limited. I have seen many examples where a parent has called the child's name again and again, interspersing this with 'no', only to find that the child shows absolutely no sign that he has heard the parent speak, and continues on, his actions unchanged.

The use of the word 'no' when meaning 'oh, don't do that' is perhaps best translated into a variety of other expressions. 'That's not nice/kind' or 'I don't like that' are some suggestions of what might be used instead. A child who has found that picking mucus out of his nose and eating it is a fascinating and tasty activity is doing something that has inherent danger only very rarely, so the problem that the parent is facing is to do with social acceptability.

There are many cultural norms that a child needs to be made aware of, and this awareness can only be developed slowly, using a number of calm, helpful, firm repeats. 'Let's do it this way' administered in a cheerful engaging way can encourage a child towards exhibiting behaviour that interfaces well in a social context.

I once saw a mother at a road crossing with a child in a buggy, and a boy, aged about three years, alongside her. I saw the boy turn to his mother and say, cheerfully, 'Just a minute, Mummy.' She waited while he ran to the litter bin that was a few yards away, deposited a wrapper in it, and ran back to her side. There was no doubt in my mind that this child had been encouraged into this behaviour pattern, rather than having been exposed to a barrage of 'no' words around the subject of litter.

There are a number of other uses of the word 'no' that might best be qualified by adding a phrase or even a sentence. 'No, not yet' indicates that the 'no' is only for now, and that the situation is likely to change. And 'no, I don't think so' has the potential of leaving dialogue open.

Appropriate containment of a child does not risk crushing or stunting that child's hunger for exploration. In fact, it enables exploration that is confident and safe. In an aura of containment, a child is free to explore and examine, knowing that the parent or carer will intervene when necessary in order to keep him and his surroundings safe.

In the waiting room of the local KwikFit, I sat and watched a man with two young boys. At first the boys entertained themselves by climbing on and off the seating, sometimes pushing behind the man when he was glancing through the newspaper. However, as time went on, their activity escalated. The man quietly made it clear that he would not allow this. The boys giggled together conspiratorially, and continued. The man took a boy under each arm and held them firmly, while chatting to them both.

The child needs adequate consistency in the messages he is given about what he should or should not do. This consistency applies to approaches from the same person, and from different people.

It is important that a child is able to observe enough of the same kind of approach coming from both of his parents. And it is helpful if the child hears his father ask 'Well, what did Mummy say?' or his mother ask 'Did you ask Daddy? What did he say?' Or indeed, either parent saying 'I'll tell you later. I'll have to check with Mummy/Daddy.' In this way he can be reassured that his parents – the two people who came together to create him – are united about his care and his direction.

'Attention-seeking' behaviour

I hear the above term used in a number of contexts in relation to children. It seems to me that behaviour that is deemed to be 'attention-seeking' is commonly viewed as being undesirable, wrong or bad. I might hear someone saying 'He is only attention-seeking. Just ignore him.' Unhelpfully, the child might merely be told 'No!' or 'Stop it!'

It is very important for children to seek attention from their parents or carers. Without sufficient interaction with the people who are responsible for them, children cannot develop and flourish.

It may well be that if a child is not receiving adequate interaction, or is perhaps receiving the wrong kind of interaction, he may go about trying to remedy this by provoking the person with whom he wants to interact. In this way, provocation can be an indirect request for a specific type of interaction. Sadly, provocation frequently invites an abrasive response, rather than being seen as a cry for help.

There is another category of provocation, and that is the one which is a test to see if the parent can provide firm containment. The child might deliberately and repeatedly present behaviour that he knows is not acceptable – specifically in order to provoke and experience firm containment from his parents. He needs to know that beyond a certain point his parents will not let this kind of behaviour continue. Through this he will develop an internalised sense of where appropriate boundaries lie.

Age gaps between siblings

If a couple wish to create a child, there are a number of considerations which might impact on their decision about when to go ahead with that plan. Chronological age of the parents, suitability of accommodation and reliability of income might be taken into account, alongside many other aspects.

Once a couple have had one child, they may decide that they want another. Here we have a situation where it is wise to consider the position of the first child, as well as revisiting practical issues in the household.

There is no simple formula for assessing the ongoing needs of the first child and how these might interface with the arrival of a potential usurper. However, we can use our intelligence to imagine the basics of what the first child will have to cope with. Then we can go on to adjust this construct to incorporate the specific needs of any particular age and stage of development of a child by the time of the pregnancy of his mother, the birth of his sibling and the ongoing presence of that sibling.

In his early life, a first child is usually the only child in his home. His access to his parents is therefore not diluted by the needs of another child. He is the one and only child. It is common for parents to feel a sense of fulfilment because they have produced a child, and their tendency to glow with pride about his existence will contribute to giving the child a good feeling about himself.

When a sibling is born, the first child is no longer 'the one and only' child. The first child has to see the mother giving to the second child all the intense focus and nursing care that used to be his alone. If, by the time the second child is born, the first child is old enough to have developed some basis of a life that does not depend entirely upon his main parent, then the second child can be welcomed as *an addition* to his life, rather than being perceived as a potential usurper and maybe even as a threat.

If the age gap between the siblings is such that the first child is still entirely dependent on the main parent, much can be done to help him with the shock of the arrival of his brother or sister. The firstborn can be gently helped to experience his sibling as a sibling, and not as a replacement for himself, but this does take a considerable amount of patience and understanding, particularly from the main carer.

During a trip to the zoo on a warm, pleasant day, I found that there were a large number of families with small children who had come to look at the animals. It was around lunchtime, and I was near the capybara enclosure when I saw a mother who had a young child and a baby. The mother was sitting on a bench, breastfeeding the baby. Her other child was a boy, who I guessed was not quite three years old. The mother was wearing shorts, and the boy stood next to her, his hand on her thigh. As he watched the passers-by, his hand moved in much the same way as I imagined that it would have done when he himself had been breastfed. It seemed as if he were an integral part of the feeding experience that was taking place.

This boy was clearly living in a situation where he knew that his place in the family had not been dislodged by the birth of his brother or sister. His sibling was an addition to his life, and was not in any way a threat.

When a baby brother or sister comes into the family, there are small children who soon wish that the baby would go away again. Some would like to parcel up the baby and send it away. Some small children have to be watched carefully in case they vent some of their upset feelings upon the defenceless baby by biting it, poking it or covering up its face. Such children may well be feeling that the baby was brought into the family as a *new, improved, version* of himself. They might feel that the parent prefers the baby and gives it more love.

If the mother is unwell during the pregnancy with her second child, a young firstborn child cannot understand why she has changed. All he knows is that she is not the same as she was, and this can be disturbing to him. If she has to be in hospital for part of the pregnancy, the stress on the firstborn is even greater, as he has to endure periods of total separation from her.

The presence of helpful extended family members or close friends who might live nearby can do much to modify the impact on a firstborn child of the changes that he has to face during his mother's pregnancy and after the arrival of his sibling.

It is not uncommon for parents to view two years as being an appropriate gap between the birth of one sibling and the next. I often hear the argument that such siblings will be close enough in age for them to grow up as friends.

However, I would like parents to consider that at two years, a child is usually at the stage where he or she needs extra help. Certainly a child of that age will require consistent patient help with his emotions, as he gradually goes through the process of expressing them and learning to name them. The presence of a new baby is a context in which many very intense emotions will be felt by the firstborn, and he will need help with every one of these. Added considerations include the fact that it is not uncommon for parents to begin 'potty training' at around the age of two years. Not only will it be difficult for a parent to remain adequately accessible for such a venture, but also it may well be hard for a child of that age to be required not to wear nappies while his new sibling is clearly wearing them all the time.

If a couple with one child does not have regular and reliable access to 'significant others' who contribute to that child's life they would be well advised to think very carefully before having an age gap of less than three years between their children. Would such a couple have sufficient inner resources to provide adequate physical and emotional sustenance to a two-year-old *and* a baby, both at the same time? Waiting longer would mean that the first child was a little more advanced in his physical and emotional development, and that some sustaining connections with the world beyond his parents and his home had been established for him. From that position he would be more able to perceive the presence of a new sibling as an addition to his life rather than someone who takes something away from him.

Considerations of 'working life' and 'career prospects' might encourage parents to think that the best way forward is to complete their family within a set time-frame. However, I would ask parents to consider very carefully where the balance might lie between the immediate needs of the very precious, longed-for, irreplaceable new human beings that they have created and concerns about adequate income or advances in personal status. Where conflict is perceived to exist between these objectives, scrupulously honest examination of all facets of the whole situation, in both a practical and an emotional sense, is of fundamental importance. Some decisions might be ones that are not ideal for anyone, but in taking everyone into account, each person benefits, as does the family unit. And it has to be recognised that some decisions might be difficult or impossible to reverse, whereas others can be reviewed along the way.

Interesting concepts …

He'll grow out of it.

Very sadly, 'growing out of it' can involve a process where the child despairs of being given an appropriate connection with a parent about whatever is troubling him at the time, so that he merely does not do whatever it is again, or does not ask about it again. To the untutored observer, it can then appear as if the child has 'grown out of' the behaviour, when in fact, the unresolved need has become buried.

Such material, when buried during the early years, is likely to re-emerge in adolescence. If so, it frequently appears in another guise, so that even if a reasonable response to that is provided, it might not meet the need that lies behind it. If unmet, the next re-emergence is likely to take place when the young person first leaves home, or gets together with his first 'proper' girlfriend. Moving in together, partnering, marrying and other such changes are other life events where buried material might come to the surface, albeit cloaked in this later theatre. Creating children, rearing them, moving home, or the death of parents provide other contexts where inner conflicts from long ago can present, but in a coded way.

'Stealing Daddy from Mummy' is a valid project when you are a little girl of three or four years old, safe in the knowledge that Mummy and Daddy understand exactly why you are feeling passionate about Daddy, want him for yourself and plan to marry him when you grow up. However, the child who has not been able to exercise safely her feeling states at that age, can become an 'adult' who finds her best friend's husband very attractive indeed… Young boys who can experiment safely with 'stealing

Mummy from Daddy' are not at risk of finding their best friend's wife intensely alluring...

The 'passionate stealing' (or having the feelings about ideas of stealing) in relation to the parent of the opposite sex when you are four years old or thereabouts is a normal, essential developmental stage. (See pages 40-42: the cameo about the girl and her parents in the Scottish Highlands.)

Some actual 'growing out of' certain states can take place along the way, if there is sufficient appropriate interaction. The child/young person remains conscious of his urges, needs and inner imperatives, and is able to make use of a range of opportunities to learn more about himself in relation to them.

Children are very resilient

The task of commenting upon this well-used statement is one which must be taken seriously. Children do have the capacity to keep struggling on *as if* they are progressing. Aided and encouraged in this, they can *seem* as if all is well enough. However, there are many situations where things are not as they seem.

Take for example a case where a child has had to endure the physical effects to his body of an accident of some kind. It may certainly be the case that the physical healing process results in his body returning to almost the same state it was in before the accident. It may also be that it is obvious that it has not, and that further help is needed. However, it may also *appear* as if all is physically well again, when it is not. Displacement of one or more of the cranial bones can frequently be missed, as can minor displacement of vertebrae. The body is adept at accommodating to such anomalies, but it can be at the cost of fully effective functioning.

The same is true of accidents and traumas to the emotions.

With help and appropriate vigilance, a place of balance can be reached again. However, a lack of balance can continue – apparent, muted or disguised.

A blanket belief in 'resilience' is not helpful, as it fails to recognise and address situations where a child requires further physical or emotional help. In cases where physical or emotional distortion is not immediately apparent, it is important to remain conscious of the possibility of its existence.

Behave yourself!

When translated, this means 'Do what suits *me*!', 'Do what *I* want!' or merely 'Shut up!'

Teaching

The word 'educate' comes from the Latin 'educo', which means 'I draw forth'. Very sadly, much of the so-called educational process does not create a setting where a child's innate intelligence is engaged in the kind of way that 'draws forth' their gifts and skills.

Quality time

What does this term actually mean? I suspect that it means different things to different people. I think that it *should* signify time that is spent together where the quality of the experience has certain special characteristics.

At best it embodies a sense of time*less*ness, where an awareness of time passing is absent. Those involved can dwell in a state where there are no barriers between them, where the flow of interaction is not impeded in any way, and trust is implicit in the relationship. It is expected that there will be a lack of interruption, or at least, no significant interruption. A feeling of 'at-one-ness' is experienced.

However, very sadly, all too often, 'quality time' might not mean that those engaged in it have experienced something of high quality.

Time spent doing something together that has been previously planned can be of high quality, but this is not necessarily the case. 'Quality time' does not mean 'activity time'. In fact, engaging in a shared activity may in some situations be an *avoidance* of participating in passage of time that is of high quality.

We should be aware of the possibility that if, in busy households, children are given focused interaction at certain times that is labelled 'quality time', it is very important that we also look at the rest of their time. If much of it is full of rushing and distraction, then there is a risk that the child develops a view that a parent is a person who has two distinct states between which there is little or no connection. At worst, there is an experience of there being two separate lives!

Part of the quality of 'quality time' depends upon the shared looking forward to it and later reminiscing about it. This valuing and treasuring of it keeps it alive and retains its meaning despite any rush and turbulence that might well be present in day-to-day life. A parent can refer to some of the special times that have been shared, thus using language that carries with it the memory of being 'at one' together. This is particularly useful when the parent is away from home, communicating with a child from a distance.

'Spoiling'

I was sitting in a waiting area looking after my baby granddaughter while my daughter had treatment for her back. Other women sitting nearby were taking a kindly interest in the baby.

Then one of them remarked to her, 'You're getting spoiled.'

I smiled and said, 'Plenty of this, at the right time and in the right way, means that she won't be trying to get it for the rest of her life, irritating people as she does so.'

Nothing else was said on the subject, and the pleasant interaction between us all continued without a break.

Final comments

When faced with the needs of a new person, through infancy, childhood and adolescence, a parent is very likely to relate to their offspring in much the same way as they themselves were related to by their own parents. After all, their parents fed and clothed them, and engineered a lifestyle in which they 'grew up', so why should anyone contemplate doing anything differently?

There are some who have an awareness that certain aspects of their childhood experience were inadequate or unpleasant. Of these, there are people who strive to ensure that their own children do not suffer similarly. However, there are others who, although realising that there were problems in their own upbringing, do not attempt to improve upon the kind of experience that they were given. Very sadly, some of these people might inflict harmful aspects of parenting upon their children in a way that can appear to be deliberate.

There are also those who are not conscious of the deleterious effects of some aspects of the parenting that they received. In general, these people are very likely to replicate most aspects of the kind of parenting that they received, helpful or unhelpful, good or bad.

We cannot create a parent who does everything right all the time. The stresses – predictable and unpredictable – that come into daily life, together with the changing face of our society, make this impossible.

The real 'perfect parent' is the 'good enough' parent – the one who has an adequate objective grasp of his strengths and his limitations, and of what life can throw into the arena of day-today living, together with an ability to make realistic plans for the future.

The good enough parent is a lifelong buddy to the new person. This buddying goes through many different phases, each appropriate to the age and stage of development of the new person.

The good enough parent reviews life regularly in the light of changed circumstances or new information, and is able to be flexible in the face of this. With a good enough parent, when things go wrong, all is not lost. In interaction with the good enough parent, a way of finding meaning and direction can be discovered or rediscovered.

The good enough parent can demonstrate true remorse when he finds that his actions have resulted in unnecessary distress coming into the life of his child.

APPENDIX

The child in therapist's clothing

I feel that it is important to consider the position of the therapist – the counsellor, the psychotherapist, the psychiatrist and the psychoanalyst, to name a few. One thing is certain – every one of these people was once a child.

Dr Ronnie Laing said as he began one of his fascinating lectures: 'The origin of the word therapist is from Greek, and it means "being with".'

Ideally we need therapists who are aware of the impact of their childhood experiences upon their capacity to mature to a fully adult state. Such self-knowledge, when combined with the theory and practice of training, is an invaluable tool in the creation of an empathic grasp of the dilemmas of the clients upon whom they depend. Self-knowledge on the part of the therapist is an integral part of an intelligent approach to the resolution of the client's problems.

Yes, we must remember that therapists depend upon their clients. Clients visit them to obtain help for the unravelling and processing of their problems, and the therapists depend upon this need for their employment.

There are therapists who learn how to dispense certain therapeutic techniques to their clients. Very sadly, such dispensing can be accompanied by a lack of any humanity and genuine warmth. If we consider whether people should be fed upon stones or upon bread, the answer is clear, and yet debate about what the therapist provides still continues. Life depends upon the interconnectedness of all living entities, and human beings are no exception to this. The invisible links that join us all must be valued and respected. Denial of them by the use of mechanistic approaches weakens and diminishes the essential links between us.

In order to 'be with' another person, we first have to be willing to know enough about ourselves and seek to continue to learn, so that we can truly be alongside the other.

I can expect that anyone who comes to me, as a therapist, for help will be struggling with certain unresolved dependent needs. It is nonsense to say to a therapist in training 'You must not let the client become dependent on you.' The very reason for the transaction between therapist and client is based on the need to examine and process unresolved dependency.

Over many years I have observed that there are some practitioners working in the field of the psychological therapies who are using their work as a kind of mask and a buffer against the disturbances in their own inner state. To them, emotional problems only exist in their clients, and can therefore be dealt with at a distance. I will give some examples.

At a full day's meeting of a prestigious association of therapists, the morning was spent listening to several speakers. The first part of the afternoon saw the participants being divided into groups, each of which went to a different room with a particular facilitator. I found myself in a group of about fifteen people, together with a facilitator who was a man in his fifties.

Not long into this session, I began to feel uncomfortable when this man spoke, apparently very knowledgeably, about the plight of many infants in a certain Eastern European country. My unease increased when it became obvious to me that he did not understand the situation about which he was speaking. Then it became clear to me that he was in the grip of the need to suppress the emotional impact of his own deprived infancy. Because of the role and responsibilities that he had accepted by being a facilitator I decided to tell him that I knew his claims were not true. I asked him to consider that he might be talking about his own problems through other people who could not represent themselves. His response was immediate, extremely loud, unbalanced and very threatening.

Amongst other things, he screamed, 'You have no right to ask me such questions!'

I replied that I had a right to ask questions, but that he did not have to answer them. That he did not have to answer them was self-evident, but I think that in the state he had entered, he had perceived me as someone who was trying to force answers from him.

Purporting to be adult anger, the powerful, all-consuming rage of a deprived infant had been presented to me. Unfortunately the therapist in which this infant dwelled was not accessible to useful discussion about his situation.

Another example involved someone who was giving a series of lectures. He was an experienced psychiatrist and psychologist. A friend of mine, who held him in high regard, had persuaded me to go to one of the lectures. That evening the subject matter was about unconditional acceptance. The lecture was of very high quality, and I found myself listening intently, considering each aspect carefully.

After about twenty minutes, the door of the room burst open, and a young man with dreadlocks entered and sat down on the floor cross-legged. He took several maps from his bag, opened one of them, laid it out on the floor and studied it. Other than the rustle of the paper, he made no sound. Everyone watched, but made no comment.

There was a pregnant silence, which was followed by...

'Get him out!' the lecturer demanded loudly to no one in particular. 'Get him out!' He was agitated and very angry.

I was sitting near the door, and my friend urged me to open it. I refused. She was clearly irritated with me, but I stood my ground. This was a lecture about unconditional acceptance of all human beings. Our visitor was a human being, and I was not going to aid any process which would lead to his exclusion.

The behaviour of the lecturer led me to conclude that the content of his lecture was a construct, and not something that he lived out in his heart and soul.

Several years later, my friend again wanted me to go with her to hear this man speak. She assured me that he had undergone four years of intense self-reflection using well-established meditative processes within a group of people who were very advanced in such matters. I decided to go along.

I was a little surprised when the speaker set up a small recording system on the chair next to his, but decided to give this no further thought. The first ten minutes of the talk demonstrated to me that this man was struggling with something so enormous that any attempt to relate to him was destined for failure. I endured the rest of the evening of the sake of my companion, but was left with an enduring image of Narcissus gazing into the lake, telling himself how wonderful he was – the speaker being the latter-day Narcissus, and the recording system being the lake.

That poor man was struggling for some sense of personal identity, and the sound of his own voice droning on and on seemed to be a calming influence upon his desperation.

A further example is from the life of friend of mine, after she had decided to train as an art therapist. Gifted in artistic expression, she had earlier attended a high-quality course at an art college. Over more recent years she had been facing problems within herself quite bravely. She felt that she was now ready to apply for the best course in art therapy that was available at that time. Part of the requirement of the two-year course was to have a one-hour session of personal therapy every week from an approved therapist.

Having secured a place on the art therapy course of her choice, she looked into the qualifications and background of a number of approved therapists. She was impressed by the profile of a woman who based her work on the principles of 'connectedness', and who gave lectures all over the world on this subject. My friend approached her, and learned that she could have weekly sessions with her, although these could not begin immediately. The college agreed to that arrangement.

After the start of the sessions, my friend, a forthright person who had worked hard to achieve a considerable amount of self-awareness and clear verbal expression, phoned me in some consternation. She wanted to talk through what had been happening in the sessions so far. From this, it seemed to me that the therapist was struggling when approached directly with valid considerations and concerns, and had said some things that were quite unbalanced. I could see that my friend was tempted to 'back off' and behave in a way she imagined that the therapist could cope with. As this would clearly be a retrograde step in her own development, I encouraged her to persist in a well-grounded and reasonable way.

The next phone call informed me that at the recent session, the therapist had become distressed, had picked up a stool, placed it in the corner of the room and had sat on it, mutely. We could only surmise that the therapist had entered a regressed state, in which she acted out a scene from when she was a small girl. Very disappointed, my friend found a different therapist to attend for the requirements of her course.

The first therapist had worn an initially invisible mask of being able to speak eloquently about connectedness. Behind that mask was a child who had been isolated into mute despair.

In contrast to these examples, I remember another lecture which I attended where the speaker, a woman, was scrupulously honest about her own reactions in situations that she described, and she was openly respectful of people who had helped to her to see herself more clearly.   She gave examples.   I was deeply impressed to learn that some of these people had been those who had been categorised as suffering from severe learning disabilities, and that she perceived and valued their wisdom with ease.

Here was someone who had a core of inner security, and who did not perceive truth to be a threat.

Donald Woods Winnicott was a very experienced hospital paediatrician, who later trained to become a psychoanalyst.   His long years of treating children in a hospital environment, together with the observations that he made of their behaviour, provided an invaluable foundation for his later work as a practising analyst. Unfettered by inner problems of his own, his therapeutic input was objective, accurate and precise, consistent and entirely human.

In order to practise as a psychoanalyst, part of the lengthy training process involves going through a full psychoanalysis oneself.   At the very least this is a recognition that in order to *be with* others in their distress, one first needs to understand one's own inner emotional structure.   However, the process of psychoanalysis is not failsafe in this respect, as Alice Miller draws to our attention in her book 'The Drama of Being a Child'.

The Dog Lead

Over many years I have pondered what to me is a central question: Does a child belong to its parents, or does it belong to society?

As far as I can tell, if a child lives with two parents (or even one) who, overall, are deemed to behave in a responsible way, then society automatically responds as if that child belongs to those people. If the child's parents are both dead, an attempt is made by certain representatives of society to find suitable substitutes. Such situations are pretty clear-cut, but there is a huge area of complexity that lies between and beyond them.

The local supermarket provides a ready context in which I can observe some of what passes between children and their parents or carers. I cannot help but be a part of it. But should this part be only a silent observation? What is my true moral place in this, and where does my responsibility to our society as a whole lie?

A recent example was the case of the boy on a post-Bulger style dog lead. I call it a 'dog lead', because that is frequently how it is used. The child is tethered rather than lovingly guided – his hand is not joined to the hand of a trusted other. I was putting my shopping through the checkout when I became aware of a boy, his mother and a trolley, two customers behind me. The boy was not yet four I would think, and although at first standing still, was emanating agitation. As his mother loaded her shopping on to the conveyor belt, he tried to put his hands where she did not want them to be. She began to tug at the lead on his wrist. Then ensued the kind of tangle that one sometimes still sees between dog and owner, where the dog ends up upside down on the ground, tangled in the lead – in a frenzy. The more frenzied this boy became, the more the mother tugged at the lead, her voice becoming louder and louder. Inwardly I cringed for this boy. The misery for him was manifest, and was bad enough; but clearly this was not the first time that this kind of thing had happened to him, and it would not be the last. What would be the long-term consequences? And, most importantly, what could I do to help? I racked my brains as I attended to my shopping, but could come up with nothing. The image has haunted me since – a 'middle-class' family out shopping for the weekly groceries…

And what about that two-year-old girl I saw, sitting in a trolley, her mother pushing? A horrible scene ensued, where the girl was offered a biscuit, but just as she reached out to take it, was ordered 'say please'. It was obvious to me that the girl was too young to understand anything but the fact that she wanted, and quite probably needed, the biscuit. Every time she reached for it, the mother snatched it away, barking 'say please'. The child's distress was mounting. I searched my mind for an appropriate way to intervene. My best attempt would be to walk past, saying something generically cheerful as an attempt to deflect or defuse the situation, but in my heart I want to sit down with any such woman and help her to look at exactly what she was saying, why she might be saying it, and what the likely consequences were of repeating it. Such behaviour can never be an integral part of a loving relationship – the kind that a child of that age, so vulnerable and entirely dependent, needs in order to be able to understand the world, and later contribute to it in a positive way.

A cluster of people at or near a trolley… Two women – mother and daughter? Deep in superficial dialogue. Two young boys holding on to the trolley, upon which a tiny baby was perched in a baby-tray in the usual near-supine posture. The older boy addresses me as if I were a close friend of the family, or at least a familiar neighbour. He and his family are strangers to me.

'I've got a baby.' His face looked tight and stressed.

'Oh yes,' I replied. 'Is it a boy baby or a girl baby?'

'It's a boy.'

There was such desperation in his voice that I could not in all conscience abandon him without having first attempted a conversation that was a validation of his attempt to relate to the world. The women took no notice. In these days of hyperawareness about potentially abusive interactions, I thought very carefully. If this child would hungrily approach me, a total stranger, for some kind of interaction, then I had to do something that would connect him to his family.

'This must be your brother,' I said, looking at the other boy at the trolley, 'and I expect that's your mummy.' Both boys nodded. I had gestured to the back of the woman who still showed no awareness of our conversation. 'Thank you for showing me your baby,' I added. 'I hope you all get the shopping you need.' I smiled and moved on, carrying with me the image of the boy who had been pitched into emptiness at this tender age. I hoped that it would be temporary. His brother had stayed largely silent, but his nodding had included him. He, of course, would be less affected, since he had his older brother for 'adult' guidance and companionship.

Many years ago I lived next door to a woman who had a small son. When he reached the age of two, and therefore showed large outbursts of feeling, she happened upon a way of 'dealing' with the noisier bursts. She would carry him upstairs, trap him on the landing behind the child gate, and then leave him, screaming desperately, alone in the house while she took the dog for a walk. I was paralysed. I could think of nothing to say or do. A baby sister was born, who could do no wrong. Some months later my son was born, and the boy next door became my little friend. He used to come round and play with me. The piano stool became a boat, and we clung to it while looking out for 'postcards' (coastguards). Our trips to the shops required some ingenuity, since local people would admire my baby son to the exclusion of my little friend. Determinedly I told them my son's name, and immediately afterwards would introduce them to my 'special friend', who glowed and chatted animatedly. I would like to meet that boy, now a man, again. I want to sit with him and think about what I was unable to prevent. I have never forgotten it. There are those who would say that *he* would have no memory of it, and so it is of no consequence. But I know that although he may not remember it in pictures, he will most certainly remember it in his emotional structure, and therefore in his reactions to events throughout his life. At the age of two, our emotions well up in us and pour out for our parents and carers to receive, understand and name for us. Much of the basis of our emotional life is laid down at that time. Why is this fundamental truth not taught in every school in the land?

Another supermarket snippet involved two women of similar age, together with a girl of around two years who was standing in the seat in the trolley, reaching out to the person who was her mother. The mother proceeded to insist to the girl that she went to her auntie, stating loudly that Auntie would be very upset if she didn't! Naturally, all the girl knew was that she herself wanted the arms of her mother before she could reach out and include another. This is such a basic reality of human development that it should hardly need to be mentioned, yet here was a 'well-intentioned' woman trying to turn upside down the natural instinct of her daughter – the very instinct which has led to human life continuing to exist at all!

In the news, we hear details of horrific cases which shock us to the core. For example, the life and death of Victoria Climbie, and the failure of the social work department to protect her and save her from her terrible fate. But where is the ongoing understanding and guidance about the intricacies of day-to-day living – living with the responsibility of nourishing society's replacements, physically, emotionally and spiritually? There are those who learn how to do this invaluable task by absorbing the truly loving approach of the mothering that they received. Among those who did not receive such care, there are many who replicate the damage that was done, by repeating it – often loudly, and verbatim – to their own young. There are others, who, because they abhor the pain and destruction that were wreaked upon them, use much of their energy to ensure that these are not passed on, or, sadly, try to behave in a 'perfect' way to everyone. They become exhausted with the effort and with the impact of what comes back in response to their approaches.

I believe that every school – and secondary schools in particular – should lay aside time each week for classes in relationship and parenting skills. There are competent guidance teachers who weave this material into their contact time, but there are also those who themselves are so damaged that they merely impose upon their unlucky charges exactly the behaviour that had distorted their own lives years earlier. There are now dolls that are programmed to behave like babies that young people can take home and 'practise looking after'. This is a very helpful and creative approach, but it represents only a fraction of the whole picture of real care and nourishment needed by the child. The term 'childcare' is used much too glibly, and can, at worst, involve no care at all. In a culture where a high proportion of all men, women and children accept that a computer cannot operate without the installation of appropriate software, it is astounding that the same basic principle is not universally applied to the rearing of society's replacements – our children. How can a fully-grown human being operate adequately without being given, along the way, the interactions that he or she needs in order to grow and mature?

In a world that desperately needs balance, wisdom and compassion as foremost qualities in its citizens, why do we fail to put sufficient of our resources into the true care of our young, so that they are nourished both emotionally and physically, and can therefore become full human beings?

And what about those who are vulnerable because of their age and deteriorating health? When my mother was assessed in her local hospital to see if she was truly capable of continuing to live on her own, I made the journey to visit her and to speak to the doctor in charge. My mother was in a single room, next to the day room where everyone gathered. There was only one other patient who could hold a conversation, and he was completely blind. I noticed a man climb behind the TV and begin to take down his trousers. A nurse called his name, and guided him to the right place. Does anyone, when rearing their young, think of what their child might have to face in old age? Kind, helpful and sensitive relating about the grasp of life requirements such as personal hygiene is essential for adequate confidence in later life, when one is when ill, ageing, or otherwise heavily dependent. If the *original* dependency in a person's life does not feel secure, then that person's ability to cope with help at a later stage will be compromised.

I recently had a phone call from a friend whose mother is now ninety. She bemoaned the fact that her mother was worrying about everything, however small. It was so clear to me that since this lady had been reared in a series of children's homes, her basic attachment needs had never been satisfied. She had never had the opportunity to develop a secure bond with one or two central people who remained accessible to her for long enough. In her infirmity she could no longer own and run her own home, and therefore was, once again, in a position where she required care. She could not conceptualise and put into words the central source of her suffering, and instead she drew her daughter into endless conversations about her worries about minutiae. In her tired mind, she could only feel all right if all her worries could be addressed. But of course that was impossible, because the real worry was unspoken by anyone. Her daughter, who longed only to have conversations with her mother that were of mutual interest, wearied in the face of this, deprived of the contact that she wanted.

A word about myself. I am, of course, not blameless. When casting my mind back through my child-rearing years, there are many evidences of my inadequacies. My pledge has always been to continue my parenting responsibilities until my death – so that anyone who was at one time a child in my care has an absolute right to approach me about anything I did or did not do that has caused him or her distress. I can never take away what happened or did not happen, but what I can do is to acknowledge and affirm the reality of the sufferer, so that he or she can continue in life, secure in the knowledge of my remorse for my earlier lack of maturity and its consequences.

The reader might think that my mind dwells solely upon misfortune and wrongness. That is not the case, and I will end with two other supermarket images.

A mother with her small daughter in the trolley strayed a little too far down the shelves for her daughter's sense of inner security.

'Mummy, don't leave me,' said the little voice.

The mother moved quickly back to the trolley and put her arm round her.

'Of course I won't, darling,' she reassured her, and she moved the trolley slowly along with her as she searched for her shopping.

The other image is of another girl, again in a trolley, this time at the checkout. She gazes happily into her mother's eyes, and her mother gazes back tenderly, reaching out and caressing her daughter's head and leaning down to kiss her forehead. The child's body radiates relaxation and contentment. I happen to know that this child was with her adoptive mother, and this gives me much hope.

So, where does the boundary lie between 'ownership' of children by their parents, and 'ownership' of children by society? The truth is that no one knows. There are situations where social workers have authority to remove children from the hands of parents who are considered to be a danger to them, but these powers are not always invoked when needed. What responsibility does each of us have, and how do we use the knowledge of it? There is little spoken in each community about such issues, yet they are fundamental to the intrinsic well-being of our society as a whole.

This essay was first published in 'On a Dog Lead' (2006).

A story for young children

A Story of Tim: The day Mummy said she and Daddy were going out in the evening.

Once upon a time, there was a boy called Tim. Tim lived with his mummy and his daddy and his little brother in a house that had an upstairs and a downstairs. The kitchen was downstairs, next to the living room, which was the place where he usually played. Sometimes Daddy would play there too, with his computer. Mummy played in the kitchen quite a lot, usually with food, but sometimes washing the clothes. And sometimes they would all play together on the floor in the living room. Tim liked that best of all.

Tim's little brother was called Jack. Tim remembered when Jack had been born. In fact, he remembered when Jack had been in his mummy's tummy. He remembered her tummy getting bigger and bigger and bigger; and he could sometimes see that the baby was moving about inside. Then one day Mummy had gone to hospital, and her tummy went small again, because Jack was outside now, and not inside her tummy. Jack had needed to have a lot of food from Mummy's breasts. Mummy explained to Tim that he, too, had needed that when he had been small like Jack. Sometimes Tim felt a little bit sad that Mummy was so busy with Jack, but he soon found that he could be part of it all. He could have a cuddle with Mummy when she was feeding Jack, or he could stroke her leg for a bit when he was playing, and that felt nice.

As Jack grew bigger, Tim found that he could help Mummy quite a bit when she was looking after him. And it was really good when Jack had started being able to play some games that Tim invented for him. Games like 'hit the balloon', 'hide in the hall', and 'bubbles in the bath'.

Mummy was Tim's mummy, and she was Jack's mummy as well. Tim and Jack could share her. Daddy was Tim's daddy, and he was Jack's daddy too. They could share him as well.

Then the wonderful day had come when Jack could go to nursery with Tim. Tim was so pleased and proud to have his very own brother at his nursery. Jack was in the special part for babies, and Tim was in the part for boys, but all the while Tim knew that Jack was there at the nursery. And when they went to nursery they always travelled together, in Mummy's car or Daddy's car.

On the days when they didn't go to nursery, there were some special days when Mummy and Daddy and Tim and Jack all went out together. Sometimes they went to visit friends, sometimes they went to visit Granny and Grandad, and sometimes they went to wonderful places to see new things. Tim liked these days very much, because everyone was together all the time. His whole family was there.

But there were one or two things that Tim sometimes didn't like as much. One of these was when Mummy and Daddy went out together and left him and Jack behind at home with a babysitter. For one thing, Tim wasn't a baby any more, and Jack wasn't really a baby either. He couldn't talk yet, but he could walk about and do all sorts of things, so he wasn't really a baby. So why did Mummy say she would get a babysitter? Of course, Tim wasn't old enough to look after Jack on his own when Mummy and Daddy went out, and there were things he needed help with himself, but he didn't need a babysitter, because he wasn't a baby. There certainly weren't any babies at his house any more.

Tim thought that when his Mummy and Daddy were out together, what he really needed was for his Auntie to come round. He liked his Auntie. She was fun, and she even looked and talked a bit like his mummy. The problem was that she couldn't always come. Mummy explained that it was because she was busy. Tim didn't always know what she was busy with, but he wished she wasn't.

One day when Mummy told Tim that she would be going out with Daddy that evening, Tim told her that he didn't like her going out with Daddy at his bedtime.

Mummy just said cheerfully, 'You'll be fine. Christine will be here while we're out.'

At least she hadn't used that word 'babysitting' thought Tim. He knew Christine quite well. She lived in a house not far away; and she had a real baby, called Mary.

'Who'll look after Mary?' he asked.

'Mary's daddy will look after her while Christine's here,' Mummy told him. 'You haven't met Mary's Daddy yet, but he's very nice, and he knows exactly how to look after Mary. She'll be fine. Of course, he can phone Christine while she's here if he needs to.'

Tim felt reassured. That sounded all right. But there was still something wrong.

'I don't want you to go out and leave me. I want to come with you and Daddy, and I want Jack to come as well,' Tim insisted. Why doesn't she understand that? he wondered to himself.

'But we're going out at your bedtime,' Mummy explained. 'If you and Jack don't go to bed at the right time, you'll be too tired to go to nursery tomorrow.'

Tim thought for a minute. He thought about the nursery, and how much he liked going there to see his friends and enjoy doing things together with the big people who helped them. He wouldn't like to be too tired to go, but he still didn't want his mummy and daddy to go out, and he said so.

'I don't want you to go out,' he said again.

Mummy sat down on one of the comfy chairs. She picked Tim up, sat him on her knee and said, 'I think we need to have a 'proper chat about this.'

It was then Tim realised that although she had said that she and Daddy were going out with Pete and Jean, who he knew quite well, he didn't know *where they were going to be*, and he didn't like that. He knew quite a lot of places now, but he had no idea where they were going to be, and that felt all wrong.

'Tell me where you're going,' he said.

Mummy cuddled him close and explained. 'We're going round to Pete and Jean's house. You know where that is, don't you? We've been there quite a few times.'

Tim nodded, and waited. He knew that his mummy hadn't finished explaining yet.

She went on. 'After that we're all going in Daddy's car to see some other friends.'

'Tell me where you're going,' Tim said again.

Mummy thought for a moment before saying, 'You know where the big shops are – the ones where we go to get shoes for you when your feet grow bigger?'

Tim nodded.

'Well, the house where we're all going is very near to those shops.'

This felt better. Tim remembered the last time he had gone for new shoes. It had been great fun. There was a very big room in the shop where children of his age tried on new shoes, and there were good things to play with in the middle of it. The nice woman had brought out lots of shoes for him to try, and Mummy had bought the blue ones he specially liked, the ones with the animal prints on the soles.

'Will you promise to go past the shoe shop on your way there?' he asked.

'Yes, of course I will,' his mummy promised, giving him another hug. 'I'll tell Daddy that's what we're going to do.'

She called out to Daddy who was busy upstairs mending a door handle. He had Jack up on the landing with him. He had put the gate at the top of the stairs so that Jack didn't fall down them while he was working.

'I've nearly finished," he called back. 'I'll be down in a minute.'

He came down with Jack tucked under one arm. Jack was waving his arms and legs around excitedly. Tim and Mummy explained their plan.

'What a good idea!' Daddy exclaimed. 'Yes, we'll be sure to go to the shoe shop.' He turned to Mummy and said, 'The shop will be shut of course, but I'll look at the window with you when we go past it, and you can tell me again about the lovely time you had there the day you and Tim got his special blue shoes.'

Mummy gave Daddy a kiss. Tim liked it when she did that. It felt all warm and cuddly to see; but he wanted to join in too, so he squeezed in between them, and they both laughed. Jack seemed quite happy under Daddy's arm, and he was still waving his arms and legs about.

Mummy thought for a minute. 'There's something else,' she said.

Tim waited expectantly.

'I got some shoes from the ladies' part of that shop once. I could put them next to your blue shoes before I go out.'

I'll put them there straight away,' Tim told her, jumping off her knee. 'Come and find them.'

Once the shoes were arranged in a neat row, Tim began to look forward to Christine coming. Perhaps she could tell him some new stories? Mummy had said that Jack would be in bed by the time Christine came. He and Christine could listen out in case Jack woke; but they could have some games and stories before it was bedtime. He could tell Christine all about nursery. Perhaps Mary would go there once she was old enough?

Tim felt excited when Mummy was making his tea. Soon he and Jack would have their bath together, with a game of bubbles, and then Mummy would put Jack in his cot. Then he would put on his pyjamas and come downstairs to wait for Christine to arrive. He expected that Mummy would be putting on some nice clothes before she went out. He liked that, too. Perhaps Daddy would be wearing his special jumper.

Once Jack was settled, the doorbell rang, and Tim and his mummy went to answer it.

'Is Mary all right?' Tim asked Christine.

'Yes, she's fine,' Christine replied, smiling at him. 'I've brought one or two things in my bag that we can do together before I tuck you up in bed,' she added.

Tim was pleased. This was all going very well. But there was something that was still bothering him. He tugged at Mummy's trousers.

'Mummy,' he said. Mummy was busy talking to Christine, so he tried again. 'Mummy!' he shouted. That worked.

'What is it?' Mummy asked.

'Can Christine phone you?' he said.

'What do you mean?' asked Mummy. Then she realised what Tim meant. 'Of course she can.' She turned to Christine and said, 'I'll give you my mobile number so you can phone me any time.'

'And Mary's daddy will phone if he wants to talk to you,' said Tim to Christine.

Christine smiled at him. 'Yes, of course he will.'

'Time to go out, Mummy and Daddy,' Tim sang as a little song.

Daddy wasn't quite ready yet, so they all waited in the hall until he came downstairs. He was wearing the nice jumper that Tim liked so much. Mummy had her pretty blouse on, and smelled very nice.

Tim hugged them both in the hall, and as he waved goodbye, he shouted, 'Don't forget the shop.'

'Come on,' he said to Christine, tugging at her hand as she

closed the door with the other hand. 'It's time to play now.'

'I have a brother,' Christine told him. 'And when we were little, we used to play together a lot of the time. Shall I tell you about some of the games we played?'

'Yes,' said Tim, pushing her down into one of the soft seats in the living room. 'And have you brought any story books in your bag?' he asked.

'Well, as a matter of fact, I have,' Christine replied. 'I've brought *The Tale of Tom Kitten* by Beatrix Potter, and *Tiny Tutak* by Hanna Wiig. My brother liked both of these stories when he was a boy like you. I used to read them again and again to him. I hope you'll like them, too. Tiny Tutak is an Inuit boy, who lived near the North Pole.'

'What's the North Pole?' asked Tim.

'I think that the next time I come when your mummy and daddy are out, I'll bring a globe with me. Then I'll be able to show you,' she replied.

'All right,' said Tim happily. Already he was looking forward to that.

By the time Christine said it was bedtime, Tim was feeling very sleepy, and he was glad to take her upstairs to show her his bed. She tucked him in and gave him a kiss.

Then he lay thinking about the interesting words that he had heard in the story about Tom Kitten. There were some long words as well, but he couldn't quite remember them. He could ask Mummy in the morning on the way to nursery, and he could tell her how Christine was going to bring a globe next time. Yes, he could remember that word – 'globe'.

The next morning, Tim heard Daddy going across the landing to the bathroom. There was no sound from Jack. He must still be asleep, he thought. And there was no sound of Mummy either.

He slipped out of bed, and ran into Mummy and Daddy's

room. Mummy was fast asleep in bed. He climbed in beside her and cuddled up to her. She didn't move, so he carefully lifted up one of her eyelids, put his mouth up against the ear that he could reach, and said, 'Time to get up now Mummy.'

Mummy opened her other eye, gave him a hug and said, 'Oh, you're so sweet. Thank you for waking me up. I'll be late for work if I stay in bed any longer. Come on, let's all get ready.' And they went together to get Jack, who was now wide awake, and was rattling the side of his cot.

At breakfast Mummy and Daddy told Tim all about how they had made sure they had gone to the shoe shop window. Tim told them how Christine used to read to her little brother, and how she had brought some of the same books to read to him.

Later, on the way to nursery with Mummy and Jack, he talked to Mummy about the long words, and she promised to speak to Christine about them.

Other reading

Babies and their Mothers   by D W Winnicott

Separation and the very young   by James and Joyce Robertson

The Drama of Being a Child   by Alice Miller

Basic Developmental Screening   by Ronald S Illingworth

A Good Enough Parent   by Bruno Bettelheim

Melanie Klein: Her Work in Context   by Meira Likierman

On a Dog Lead   by Mirabelle Maslin

Carl and other writings   by Mirabelle Maslin
Final essay: What is going wrong?   by W N Taylor

* * * * * *

Frog and Toad are Friends   by Arnold Lobel

The Penguin and the Vacuum Cleaner   by Carolyn Sloan

Tracy   by Mirabelle Maslin

The Demon Headmaster   by Gillian Cross

Matilda by Roald Dahl

The Witches by Roald Dahl

Titles from Augur Press

Beyond the Veil

ISBN 0-9549551-4-5 £8.99

Fay

ISBN 0-9549551-3-7 £8.99

Emily

ISBN 978-0-9549551-8-2 £8.99

a trilogy by Mirabelle Maslin

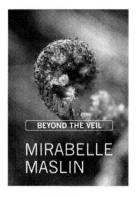 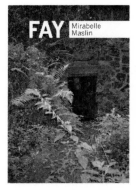 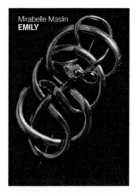

Spiral patterns, a strange tape of music from Russia, a 'blank' book and an oddly shaped walking stick ...

Fay suffers from a mysterious illness. In her vulnerable state, she is affected by something more than intuition ...

Emily meets Barnaby. Sensing that they have been drawn together for a common purpose, they discover that each carries a crucial part of an unfinished puzzle from years past ...

Order from your local bookshop, amazon.co.uk or the Augur Press website at www.augurpress.com

The Fifth Key by Mirabelle Maslin

ISBN 978–0–9558936–0–5   £7.99

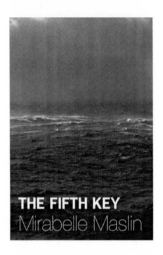

Soon after Nicholas' thirteenth birthday, his great-uncle John reveals to him a secret – handed down through hundreds of years to the 'chosen one' in every second generation. John is very old. His house has long since fallen into disrepair, and as Nicholas begins to learn about the fifth key and the pledge, John falls ill. Facing these new challenges and helping to repair John's house, Nicholas begins to discover his maturing strengths.

The unexpected appearance of Jake, the traveller whom Nicholas has barely known as his much older brother, heralds a sequence of events that could never have been predicted, and a bond grows between the brothers that evolves beyond the struggles of their ancestors and of Jake's early life.

Order from your local bookshop, amazon.co.uk or the augurpress website at www.augurpress.com

The Candle Flame by Mirabelle Maslin

ISBN 978-0-9558936-1-2   £7.99

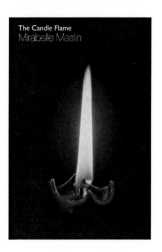

One dark winter's night, an unseen force attacks Molly, leaving her for dead. On their return from snaring rabbits, her husband, Sam, and his brothers, James and Alec, discover her, and slowly nurse her back to life. But she cannot speak. Determined to avenge Molly and help her to regain her voice, the brothers search for clues. Could her affliction be due to a curse? The birth of Sam and Molly's son, Nathan, raises questions about his ancestry. Who was Molly's father, and how did he meet his end? Might there be a connection between violent events of long ago and Molly's present state?

Order from your local bookshop, amazon.co.uk or the augurpress website at www.augurpress.com

Titles from Augur Press

Self-help novellas
by Mirabelle Maslin

Miranda	£6.99	978-0-9558936-5-0
Lynne	£6.99	978-0-9558936-6-7
Field Fare	£6.99	978-0-9558936-8-1

Poetry

The Poetry Catchers
   by Pupils from Craigton Primary
   School
	£7.99	978-0-9549551-9-9

Poems of Wartime Years by W N Taylor	£4.99	978-0-9549551-6-8
The Voice Within by Catherine Turvey	£5.99	978-0-9558936-3-6
Now Is Where We Are by Hilary Lissenden	£6.99	978-0-9558936-7-4

Trilogy by Mirabelle Maslin

Beyond the Veil	£8.99	978-0-9549551-4-4
Fay	£8.99	978-0-9549551-3-7
Emily	£8.99	978-0-9549551-8-2

Other novels

One Eye Open: Can a Dolphin Save the World? by Steve Cameron	£7.99	978-0-9571380-1-8
The Candle Flame by Mirabelle Maslin	£7.99	978-0-9558936-1-2
Letters to my Paper Lover by Fleur Soignon	£7.99	978-0-9549551-1-3

For children and young people

The Supply Teacher's Surprise by Mirabelle Maslin	£5.99	978-0-9558936-4-3
Tracy by Mirabelle Maslin	£6.95	978-0-9549551-0-6
The Fifth Key by Mirabelle Maslin	£7.99	978-0-9558936-0-5

Eating disorder
Size Zero and Beyond: £13.99 978-0-9571380-0-1
A personal study of anorexia
nervosa by Jacqueline M Kemp

Hemiplegia
Hemiplegic Utopia: Manc Style £6.99 978-0-9549551-7-5
by Lee Seymour

Sexual Abuse
Carl and other writings £5.99 978-0-9549551-2-0
by Mirabelle Maslin

Health
Mercury in Dental Fillings £5.99 978-0-9558936-2-9
by Stewart J Wright
Lentigo Maligna Melanoma: £5.99 978-0-9558936-9-8
A sufferer's tale
by Mirabelle Maslin

Miscellaneous
On a Dog Lead £6.99 978-0-9549551-5-1
by Mirabelle Maslin

Ordering:
Online   www.augurpress.com

By Post   Delf House, 52, Penicuik Road, Roslin,
Midlothian EH25 9LH   UK

Postage and packing: £2.00 for each book, and add £0.75p for each
additional item.

Cheques payable to Augur Press. Prices and availability subject to
change without notice. When placing your order, please indicate if
you do not wish to receive any additional information.

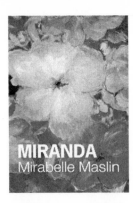
MIRANDA
Mirabelle Maslin

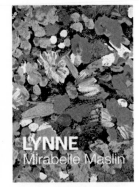
LYNNE
Mirabelle Maslin

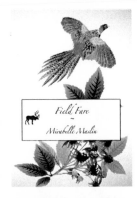
Field Fare
~
Mirabelle Maslin

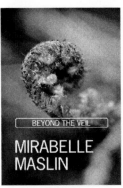
BEYOND THE VEIL

MIRABELLE MASLIN

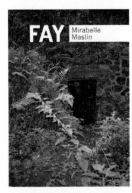
FAY Mirabelle Maslin

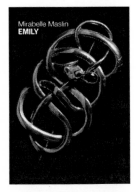
Mirabelle Maslin
EMILY

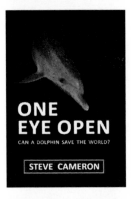
ONE EYE OPEN
CAN A DOLPHIN SAVE THE WORLD?

STEVE CAMERON

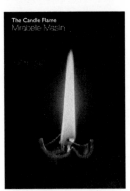
The Candle Flame
Mirabelle Maslin

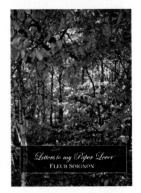
Letters to my Paper Lover
FLEUR SOIGNON

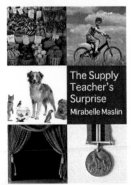
The Supply Teacher's Surprise
Mirabelle Maslin

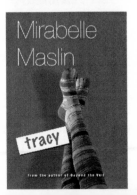
Mirabelle Maslin

tracy

from the author of Beyond the Veil

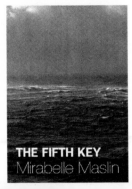
THE FIFTH KEY
Mirabelle Maslin

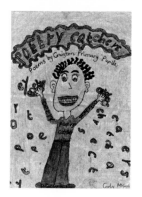

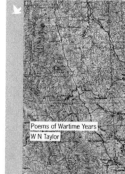

Poems of Wartime Years
W N Taylor

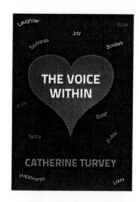

Laughter Soul
Joy
Sadness Smiles

THE VOICE
WITHIN

Pain

Fear Pride

CATHERINE TURVEY

Happiness Love

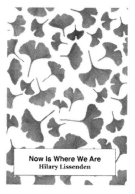

Now Is Where We Are
Hilary Lissenden

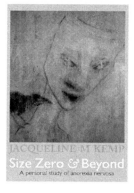

JACQUELINE M KEMP
Size Zero & Beyond
A personal study of anorexia nervosa

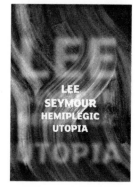

LEE

LEE
SEYMOUR
HEMIPLEGIC
UTOPIA

UTOPIA

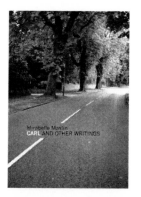

Mirabelle Maslin
CARL AND OTHER WRITINGS

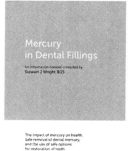

Mercury
in Dental Fillings

An information booklet compiled by
Stewart J Wright BDS

The impact of mercury on health,
Safe removal of dental mercury,
and the use of safe options
for restoration of teeth

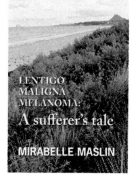

LENTIGO
MALIGNA
MELANOMA:
A sufferer's tale

MIRABELLE MASLIN

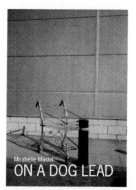

Mirabelle Maslin
ON A DOG LEAD